THE
CANTIN
KETOGENIC
DIET

For Cancer, Type I Diabetes
& Other Ailments

Elaine Cantin

D0958657

LCCN: 2012909945

ISBN-13: 978-1477567593

ISBN-10: 1477567593

Editors: Katherine Cantin, Gillie Moorhawk, Jill Ross

Cover: Michele Pare

DISCLAIMER

All the ideas, concepts, and the opinions expressed here in this book are intended to be used for educational purposes only.

This book is supplied on the understanding that the author is providing her personal experience, along with a summation of published scientific and medical research, and is not rendering any kind of medical advice. This book is not intended to replace any medical advice, nor diagnose, or treat any disease, illness, condition, or injury. It is extremely important that before starting any diet program, including this book's program, that you consult with a licensed physician and follow this diet program under the medical supervision of your healthcare provider.

This program is recommended to be used in combination with medical treatment from your healthcare provider, not instead of it.

The author and the publisher claim no responsibility to any person or entity for any liabilities, damage, and loss caused or alleged to be caused directly or indirectly as a result of the personal use, personal interpretation, and personal application of the material in this book.

By continuing to read this book you are assumed to have read and agreed to this disclaimer.

DEDICATION OF THIS BOOK

To Drs. John M. Freeman and to Jeanne Go for all their kindness and hard work with the little sick children.

Dr. Freeman... you made a difference in my life when everyone treated me like I was crazy when they did not understand what I was talking about. You, on the other hand...you took the time and wrote to me that you thought I was "perceptive." You gave me motivation to continue and to ignore the negative. You taught me important things that helped me save my life and write this book. You're a special person.

Dr. Go, first you saved my son's life...there are just no words good enough to describe you. Then, you stood by us and you were open-minded about food, ketogenic diets, and even fasting. When I think about you, I just feel love and gratitude.

CONTENTS

Preface

There are so many threads that came together and led to the creation of this diet. My son's diagnosis with type I diabetes in 1999 was the first step in a long journey that has spread over the last thirteen years. How was I to know that my dedication in trying to understand my son's condition, would lead, so many years later, to a life-saving cure for my own recurrence of aggressive breast cancer, and then in turn this would lead me to understand how to get my son off insulin? How was I to know that going through all this would also help my sister after emergency brain surgery? Coincidence? I don't think so. So many pieces of the puzzle all came together to create a new picture that I believe can help so many people.

This book is the summation of research that came directly from my heart and culminated in the creation of my own variation on the traditional ketogenic diet. I want to share this information with all of you.

Acknowledgments

There are many people who were essential steps on this journey of discovery for me. Thank-you notes go, in no particular order, to the following people:

- Johns Hopkins Medical Center in Baltimore, Maryland, and its doctors for their work and research with the ketogenic diet.

- Dr. John M. Freeman for his book, *The Ketogenic Diet,* and also for being kind when I e-mailed him about my son. He was one of the few people who could understand what I was talking about when I linked epilepsy with type I diabetes. He is part of the reason I am alive today and the best teacher anyone could have.

- Dr. William B. Coley, whose research on injecting toxins to induce fever and produce cancer remission helped point me in the right direction to get rid of my own cancer tumor recurrence.

- Dr. Jerry R. Gerson, for being kind and a friend to me when my son was first diagnosed with Type I diabetes and for helping me when he was resisting insulin.

- My family and dear friends, who were there for me and supported me when I was diagnosed with breast cancer. Especially my daughter's and my son's support that meant so much to me.

- Monique Ricard, who cured her stage 4 terminal breast cancer naturally and inspired me to do the same.

- My friend, Gilli Morehawk, who went through breast cancer too and helped me with this book.

- My guardian angels who have led me every step of the way.

- The movie producer Jim Abrahams for his inspirational movie *First Do No Harm* which described his search for a cure for his son Charlie's epilepsy.

- Suzanne Somers and her book *Knockout* for teaching me about the importance of balancing hormones and the importance of spices, herbs, supplements, vitamins, and organic foods to boost the immune system. Also for making me aware of the work of such doctors as Dr. Stanislaw Burzynski, Dr. Jonathan Wright, Dr. Russell Blaylock, and Dr. Nicholas Gonzalez, who are all pushing forward the research and knowledge for treatments for all types of cancer.

- Dr. Robert Coleman Atkins, for teaching me you can also get the body to produce ketones with the combination of high protein and high fat and very low carbohydrates. His work helped me to come up with a diet that is ketogenic without using any of the major allergens.

- Dr. Mary Newport, for her work with ketones, coconut oil, and Alzheimer. Her work helped me with my sister after brain surgery.
- Last but certainly not least: Dr. Jeanne Go, who saved my son's life when she diagnosed him with type I diabetes in 1999. You are forever in my heart, and I truly believe you are an angel on hearth.

CHAPTER ONE

Brief History for Epilepsy & Type I Diabetes

Let's start with some history, going back in time to the early 1900s, and focusing on the traditional ketogenic diet and "the Allen starvation treatment"[1].

The traditional ketogenic diet- which mimics fasting/starvation- was used to treat epilepsy before epileptic drugs were invented. The Allen starvation treatment was used to treat Type I Diabetes, before the discovery of insulin.

It appears from history that the Allen starvation Treatment was the dawn of the ideas of the traditional ketogenic diet.

The book *Ketogenic Diet A Treatment For Children And Others With Epilepsy*[2] explains the following:

A) *Fasting has been used since biblical times as a treatment for seizures and epilepsy. Renewed interest for fasting came after a 1921 American Medical Association convention. There, a well-*

---

known doctor spoke about fasting and the successful treatment of severe epilepsy. That doctor was a pediatrician in New York named Rawle Geyelin. His friend's child's case was cited. The child was ten years old and had been having mostly continuous seizures for four years. Under the care of Dr. Hugh Conklin, the child was put on a fasting treatment. At first the fast lasted fifteen days, then some time for foods, and then fasting again. Dr. Geyelin reported that this resulted with the seizures stopping after the second day on the fast and the child being seizure-free for the following year. Two other patients of Dr. Conklin were also reported as being seizure-free for two and three years after treated with fasts. Geyelin also reported that he used fasting to treat twenty-six of his own epileptic patients with eighteen of the twenty-six showing significant improvements. This was the first time in American history that the benefits of fasting for epilepsy were reported. Later, Dr. William Lennox linked Conklin's work with fasting to the origin of the ketogenic diet.

B) *The link with Johns Hopkins Hospital: the father of Dr.Conklin's ten year-old epileptic patient was Charles Howland, a wealthy New York attorney. The child's uncle was Dr. John Howland, professor of pediatrics at the Johns Hopkins Hospital and director of the newly opened Harriet Lane Home for Invalid Children at Johns Hopkins Hospital in Baltimore. In 1919, Dr. John Howland was given funding by his brother to do some scientific research on his son's treatment. A laboratory was established for this. After hearing reports from Dr. Geyelin that fasting could cure seizures, various researches all over the US started.*

C) *During this same period, work was being done to try to understand type I diabetes. Doctors wanted to know why the body was unable to burn glucose and to understand its consequences, such as dehydration, chemical imbalance, comas, and even death. It is very important to note here that it is also mentioned in* Ketogenic Diet: A Treatment For Children And Others With Epilepsy *that these consequences with type I diabetes did not occur with starvation or the ketogenic diet because the glucose is restricted.*

D) *Discovery of the traditional ketogenic diet: An article from Wilder was published in 1921 and it suggested a diet high in fats and low in carbohydrates to produce ketogenesis. In 1924, Peterman from the Mayo Clinic reported on this "ketogenic diet". The diet was made of 1 gram of protein per kilogram of body weight for children, and it was less for adults: a maximum of 10 to 15 grams of carbohydrates per day. The remaining daily calories came from fat. A person's daily caloric intake was calculated based on the "basal metabolic rate plus 50 percent." This is similar to what is still being used today.*

***

As mentioned previously, there was some research being conducted on type I diabetes running parallel to epilepsy research. Here is some historical information for the low-carbohydrate diets used to treat diabetes before the discovery of insulin, like the Allen starvation treatment[3] . It is to be noted that even after the discovery of insulin, diet was and still is an important part of diabetes maintenance.

Per the ADA and a published article titled "Rethinking the Triad of Diabetes in the New Millennium"[4]...

> There were only a few known cases of type 2 diabetes in the past, as compared to now, and type I diabetes was extremely rare. The only treatment options for type I diabetes before the discovery of insulin was diet and exercise, but this usually would not keep the patient alive for very long. One example of such diets was the Allen starvation diet that was used from 1910 to 1921. These diets were said to have a "starvation approach" because they used fasting until "glucosuria" cleared, and then introduced moderate quantities of protein and fat with a low carbohydrate intake. They also had to keep the patients on a very low daily caloric intake -like around 400 calories per day- which was borderline starvation, in order to prevent the blood glucose from going up to dangerous levels. On the type of diet they were feeding the patients, they could hardly feed them without the blood glucose going up.
>
> Insulin was available for treating type I diabetes after 1922, but only in short supply and purity was an issue. Methods for testing blood glucose were not what they are today

and urine testing was used to help with insulin dosage. Even after the discovery of insulin, diet had to be taken into account, as shown by a book by Dr. Joslin called A Diabetic Manual for the Mutual Use of Doctor and Patient[5] (this book was used before and for a while after the discovery of insulin). Still today, treating type I diabetes with diet and insulin is hard to manage and often leads to complications.

***

THE CANTIN KETOGENIC DIET

CHAPTER TWO
How Fasting/Starvation and
The Ketogenic Diet Work

Per the book "Ketogenic Diets,"[6] we learn the following:

A) The standard American diet is composed of approximately 50 to 60% carbohydrates and the rest is composed of protein and fat. On this type of diet, the body burns glucose as its main source of fuel for energy.

B) The body can store supplies of glucose for only up to thirty-six hours. Therefore, during fasting or starvation, the body burns body fat for its source of fuel for energy after the glucose supplies have been depleted. That is a survival mechanism. However, if you fast for too long and there is no more fat left, then the body starts burning muscles. This can affect a person's energy, health and can cause death.

C) In contrast to standard American diet, the traditional ketogenic diet is very low in carbohydrate intake. Once the glucose supplies have been depleted, the body starts burning fat coming from food as a source for fuel for energy. Thus, this diet mimics fasting or starvation in the way that you are burning fat for energy, but unlike fasting or starvation, you will not compromise your health because you are eating and will not run out of fat. Unlike fasting or starvation, being on a ketogenic diet for a long period of time will not cause death.

D) When there is no glucose, or when glucose is restricted enough, the fat is not burned entirely and a residue called ketone bodies is left. The ketone bodies that are left are beta-hydroxybutyric acid and acetoacetic acid.

The traditional ketogenic diet is composed of the following food combination: high fat, very low carbohydrate and low protein.

From Dr. Atkins' book Dr. Atkins' Diet Revolution,[7] we learn that we can also produce a ketogenic diet with the following food combination: high fat, high protein, and low carbohydrate.

One of the major sources of fat in these diets is dairy. Dairy is also a major food source in the diets listed previously from Dr. Joslin and from Dr. Allen for managing type I diabetes.

***

CHAPTER THREE
Benefits of a Ketogenic Diet

Why can a ketogenic diet be good for cancer, type I diabetes and other ailments? A diet that is ketogenic has three ketone body sources [8]:
A) BHB or beta-hydroxybutyrate (over 75%)
B) acetoacetate (less than 25%); and
C) acetone, which is a derivative of acetoacetate (approximately 2%).

A)
The major source of ketone bodies is BHB and it is linked to increase of glutathione (GHS), which is a major antioxidant in the body, master detox and anti-inflammatory. It is also linked to the decrease of reactive oxygen species (ROS). See the article "The ketogenic diet increases mitochondrial glutathione levels"[9] for more details on this.

Regarding the importance of glutathione, there are videos from Dr. Herbert Nagasawa[10] and Dr. Mark Hyman[11] that provide more details on the importance of glutathione. They explain the benefits of glutathione, such as helping "maintain cellular redox homeostasis," which means it helps maintain the body pH to normal; transporting

────────────────

amino acids to the cell; and carrying oxygen to the cell. That is important because per Dr. Otto Warburg, cancer cells grow in an environment without oxygen and by fermentation of sugar.[12]

It also has to do with hormonal levels that are responsible for body regeneration, muscle growth, fat burning, tissue repair, strength and insulin levels.[13] [14] [15]

B)

The second major source of ketone bodies is acetoacetate and research shows it reduces cancer cells growth (see the article titled "Acetoacetate reduces growth and ATP concentration in cancer cell lines which over-express uncoupling protein 2.") [16]

C)

The last source of ketone bodies is acetone. Acetone is a derivative of acetoacetate and is also a symptom of disease, like a viral infection that causes fever, vomiting, and diarrhea. The fever and the vomiting may increase and if it happens, it becomes a closed- meaning a cycle of more vomiting, more acetone, more fever, and more vomiting until the closed is stopped.[17]

According to the definition of Ketonuria on Wikipedia, "there is a positive relationship between the presence of ketonuria after fasting and positive metabolic health." [18] Research presented in "Ketonuria after Fasting May be Related to the Metabolic Superiority" [19] also stresses this.

Some food or supplements that are included in my diet in this book also directly increase glutathione; for examples, proteins, some vegetables, curcumin, as observed by research "Curcumin treatment alleviates the effects of glutathione depletion in vitro and in vivo: therapeutic implications for Parkinson's disease explained via in silico studies," [20] N-acetylcysteine (NAC), [21] and EGCG, found in green tea. [22] [23]

Per the article titled "Theoretical Basis of the Ketogenic Diet," [24] *ketone bodies have a sedative effect and an appetite-suppressing effect.* That is positive for those wishing to lose weight, and at the same time it is also involved in preventing cachexia- meaning the reduction of weight loss in what is called the "wasting away" process in cancer. That is also very positive. See the following research paper for more details: "Reduction of weight loss and tumour size in a cachexia model by a high fat diet."[25]

CHAPTER FOUR

TYPE I DIABETES
A Mother is the Necessity for Invention

My journey started fifteen years ago when my beautiful son was born in February 1997, whole and healthy and perfect. I fell in love with him immediately.

One weekend in January 1999, just before his second birthday, I felt there was something wrong with him. He was just lying on the couch very quietly. It was not like him at all; normally he was a very active little boy. At first I thought maybe he was coming down with a cold. The cold did not come and he had no fever. On Monday morning when he was still no better, I called his pediatrician's office and asked them to take him in between patients because I knew something was wrong with him. They squeezed him in that day, because Dr. Go never refuses any kids - thank god for her open door policy. When she saw him and put her stethoscope on his heart, she felt something was wrong right away. Very calmly she said that my son's heartbeat and breathing suggested something was wrong and he might have swallowed something that he'd picked up at home; a toy or something like that and she was going to hospitalize him right away to make sure he got the best care. The hospital could do all the necessary tests.

I know Dr. Go saved my son's life. The hospital doctors told me later that if I hadn't taken him to the hospital that day he would probably have been dead within twenty-four hours. Dr Go is an angel and so special and I'm so grateful I found her to take care of my kids. When I was searching for a doctor her staff recommended her so highly to me and they were right. Her young patients all love her as she comes into the exam room with a stethoscope around her neck, with Barney and other stuffed animals tied to it with Velcro and she would push a rattan basket with toys falling down around it and playing nursery songs. It was like magic for kids when she would walk in the exam room. Everyone adores her.

At the hospital they did blood tests and X-rays, and then Dr. Go broke the news to us that my precious boy had type I diabetes. They started him on an insulin drip and he was taken by ambulance to the children's intensive care unit at St. Mary's Hospital in West Palm Beach, Florida.

His blood glucose was in the 700s when the normal range should be 70-110 mg/dl. The specialist told us that he would be critical for the next forty-eight hours and that even if he survived, he might have brain damage because of the "DKA" (diabetic ketoacidosis).

David was already potty trained so I didn't notice if he was urinating more than normal; that's one of the few early signs of diabetes along with being thirsty all the time.

Not surprisingly, I was a basket case. My perfect little baby was fighting for his life and we were all in shock. For three days and nights, I did not sleep and I could not eat. I stayed with him every moment and wished it could be me when he was crying because they were hurting him as by drawing blood samples, and pricking his fingers to test his glucose level.

When he was sleeping, I just kept praying he would pull through. When I was told by the nurse that I had to leave for one hour during the morning and for one hour at night during staff changes, due to construction and for the staff not having a private room to discuss patients...I started crying and told the nurse there was no way I would leave my child alone when he needed me most. I said that I had just read the Patients' Bill of Rights and I was allowed to refuse treatment at any time for my child, so if she wanted to enforce this ridiculous rule with me, then I would refuse treatment for my child for one hour in the morning and one hour at night and I would hold my child in my arms in the waiting room along with his insulin bag, heart monitor, and with all the other stuff he was hooked up to.

They relented after that and allowed me to stay with David all the time. Because I was there all the time I soon realized they had also made an error in ordering lab works for my son and someone was coming to draw blood in error every half hour. I was not going to leave him alone.

Fortunately, after fourty-eight hours he was released from ICU and there was no sign of any brain damage from this trauma.

After a day or two in intermediate care, the doctor said I could take him home as soon as they were confident I could take care of him. I had to demonstrate that I could use the blood glucose meter to test his blood glucose as needed, give him his insulin injections, and draw insulin from the vials correctly not mixing up the long acting and short acting insulin, and without any air bubbles in the syringe.

I was desperate to get David home, but they didn't have any staff who could teach me to use the particular meter that the doctor prescribed and they refused to let me go until I could demonstrate how that particular meter worked. Right away, in desperation, I looked at the meter brand and called the company's 800 number. I burst into tears as I told the woman on the line that she needed to teach me how to use that meter so I could take my child home from the hospital. That wonderful woman was so kind to me and she talked me through the process until I knew exactly how to do it. Once I'd showed the nurses how the meter worked by demonstrating it on myself, I showed them I could draw insulin and I could give injections, I finally could take my boy home.

The first time I gave him an injection was so hard. I wanted to cry and wished he didn't have to go through this but I had no choice, and neither did David. Insulin injections would be a daily occurrence for us from then on and we all just had to get used to it.

It was the thought of him spending the rest of his life enduring daily insulin injections and the risk of the many complications from diabetes that drove me to find out everything I could to help him. I was heart-broken that my beautiful boy was going to suffer this fate and determined to find some way to help him recover. Even though my mind knew that diabetes was a life-long condition, my heart was telling me there had to be some other way. As I drove home from the hospital, I remember thinking that at least it was not cancer and I would still have him in my life…

***

When racking my brain to find out what happened that was different that could have caused him to be diagnosed with type I diabetes, I came up with the following list: about seven months prior to diagnosis he was vaccinated for hepatitis B; about four months before diagnosis, he was stung by bumble-bees, about a month prior to diagnosis he was sick with a virus, and about one or two months prior to diagnosis I had stopped boiling water for him and had started giving him water from the tap.

I started learning all I could about Type I diabetes and what I could do to try to help my son. I noticed that when I cooked breakfast for him- egg, potatoes, and sausage, cooked in extra-virgin olive oil- he would need approximately one-third less insulin than when his father cooked the exact same breakfast in butter. I also noticed that if he had a meal cooked with a lot of butter, he would need three to five times more insulin.

I tried to talk to his endocrinologist about it but I was treated like I was crazy and brushed off. However, Dr. Go told me that if a mother tells her that dairy products hurt her child, she believes it. She sent me with David to see a doctor for allergies and my son tested negative for that particular test. The Doctor told me that he had never heard that a food like dairy would cause blood glucose to go up, but if that was my experience, I should take my child off dairy. He also told me that if something in the diet causes an allergic reaction and is completely removed, later a very small amount can cause a more severe allergic reaction. We also tried the dairy-free products to find out if it was intolerance, but those would also cause an adverse reaction in my son's body, which indicated he had an allergy and not an intolerance to dairy. I do not think that my son was tested for beef protein allergy. I cannot remember for sure.

Per the allergist's instructions, I started writing down everything David ate and keeping track of his blood glucose fluctuation for different foods. We kept him off dairy as much as we could, though I found that when I tried replacing cow's milk with soy milk, David had the same negative reaction to it. Dr. Go told me that most of her patients who were allergic to lactose were also allergic to soy.

After I saw how my son was reacting so badly to milk, I found I could not drink it myself anymore. I had been a milk drinker all my life but now it disgusted me. I also took my daughter off cow's milk for fear that she could also get type I diabetes from it. I learned to read labels and watch out for "hidden" cow's milk names such as casein, caseinate, whey, whey protein, lactose, lactate, lactalbumin, milk enzymes, milk protein, curds, flavouring and natural flavour. Lactic acid can be a possible source of dairy as well.

NOTE: When my son was a newborn and before he had Type I diabetes, I had noticed that he had a problem with dairy-based formula. He would throw up a little after his bottle. He was my second child and my daughter did not have that problem, so I asked his doctor at the time about it. I was told that if he could tolerate the cow's milk formula it was better to keep him on it, as it had more nutrients. I have a history of various food allergies and passing out as a teenager due to hypoglycemia, and my mom was also diagnosed with some form of intolerance to glucose. So it seems like some kind of food sensitivity runs in my family. I read an article called: *"Children's Memorial Food Allergy Study: Addressing Major Questions about Food Allergies in Children."*[26] This research suggests that allergies are linked to genetics and environmental factors. When I was pregnant with my son, I also remember craving milk.

Approximately a year after David was first diagnosed with Type I diabetes, he became very sick with fever, severe vomiting, and elevated ketone in his urine. Dr. Go hospitalized him as a precaution so he would not become dehydrated. He was hooked up to sugar-free I.V. fluid. I stayed at the hospital around the clock to take care of him, so I know everything he ate and drank. At first he couldn't hold any solid foods and I gave him diet ginger ale. An acquaintance of my sister, who was a type I diabetic before he had a pancreas and liver transplant, had told her that the only thing that would drop his blood glucose when his body was resisting insulin, was drinking a hot cup of chicken broth and a cup of ginger ale immediately afterwards. He had learned this from other diabetics.

Since the doctors advised to try to always have no ketone for a diabetic, I kept checking his urine with urinalysis testing strips for presence of ketone. He was showing large ketone values in his urine.

Gradually, his blood sugar kept dropping nonstop. I had to keep giving him sugar pills and regular ginger ale to bring his blood sugar back up to normal and he still kept dropping. I kept having to decrease his insulin dose. When he started eating, all he wanted to eat was the home-cooked ham brought from home (i.e.: protein), so that is what I gave him.

By the time David was released from the hospital, his body started working again and he was *completely off insulin* for three full days. He could eat and drink anything and the blood sugar would stay in normal range without any insulin at all. It was like he was cured. At first he had the high ketone in the urine; it gradually decreased to none after the third day and he then started needing the insulin again when the ketone became negative. At the time, I did not even think about linking ketone with his situation. I was just so terribly sad that he had to go back on insulin and I so wanted to understand what had happened to get him off insulin. I kept thinking that there had to be a logical explanation.

When I spoke to his endocrinologist about it, I was just told it was a fairly common occurrence for a newly diagnosed diabetic patient to have a 'honeymoon-phase' when they suddenly don't need insulin any more, just before the cells all die.

Years later, I found out, thanks to Dr. John M. Freeman, information that makes a lot more sense to explain this. It was known in the medical field since the era of the "Allan starvation treatment" that fasting (starvation) would bring down the blood glucose to normal and would decrease the need for insulin. Since my son had a high fever, was fasting, and had ketosis (per the tests I did), my son's experience is just another proof that this early observation was accurate and made sense. Again, thanks to Dr. Freeman, I found out this was the treatment for type I diabetes before insulin was discovered, and this was also sort of the dawn for the basis of the ketogenic diet.

However, at the time this happened, I had never heard of: the book *Breakthrough* (by Thea Cooper and Arthur Ainsberg), the ketogenic diet, nor the Allen "starvation" treatment for type I diabetes, and I had no clue it was known that fasting decreased the need for insulin.

It was only years later (thanks to Dr. Freeman) that I found out that before insulin was discovered, they used to starve type I diabetics to keep them alive. After the starvation/fasting period, they would put them on the diet described in the "Allen Starvation Treatment." This diet contained only about four hundred calories per day.

An important quote from Dr. Allen:

"The functional character of the pancreatic disturbance in many or most cases of human diabetes is worthy of all emphasis. A functional disease must be curable"[27] ~Frederick M. Allen

***

At the time, I kept trying to figure out what had happened. Thoughts and facts kept whirling around my brain: the foods he ate, the things he drank, and the pattern of ketone values in his urine and the variation in his blood tests. I kept thinking that there had to be a logical explanation for all this and just kept turning it over and over in my mind… Then, approximately a year after that, by pure chance, I just happened to watch a movie on national TV about a diet used to treat epileptic children.

The movie was called First Do No Harm and it not only touched my heart deeply, but it also struck me due to the similarities I found with my son's situation -working so hard to monitor and balance his food and only being allowed to eat certain things. I became curious about the diet- especially the part about having to keep the kids showing a high level of ketone in the urine to stop the seizures. The hard work with the diet/food also really resonated with me. The movie did not go into many details;

_____

it was more to make this diet known. So I started looking into the ketogenic diet and all the pieces of the puzzle fell into place. Suddenly it all became clear in my mind what had happened to my son; how he could get off the insulin and why his body started working again…

Just like the kids who were put on the ketogenic diet at Johns Hopkins, David's body went into large ketone because he had a fever and he was not eating anything. This signalled his body to stop using the sugar as fuel for energy, and instead, his body switched to burning fat for energy. Burning fat led to a different internal physiological process and this somehow decreased the need for insulin and allowed him to be off insulin completely for full three days, until the ketone levels dropped to zero and he needed to be put back on insulin. I was there with him at all times, monitoring his blood glucose, checking ketone levels, giving insulin, and making sure the blood glucose was kept as close as possible to normal range. Dr. Go had hospitalized him and requested sugar free I.V. so he had fluid to make sure he would not get dehydrated. I was giving him the diet ginger ale and he had no sugar (except for when the blood glucose started dropping).

I then bought the book *The Ketogenic Diet.*[28] by Dr. John M. Freeman to get even more details about the ketogenic diet. I read this book so many times and found so many similarities with my son's situation. I am extremely grateful to Dr. Freeman for this book and all the details he provided.

I tried to talk about this ketogenic diet but nobody would listen and the medical establishment tells you that you **must** avoid ketone due to the deadly danger of diabetic ketoacidosis (DKA) that most people confuse with ketosis during either starvation/fasting or while on a ketogenic diet.

Let me point out again here what I pointed out earlier in this book and referenced under note number 2 from the book *The Ketogenic Diet*: *In diabetic ketoacidosis, the inability to burn glucose leads to exceedingly high levels of blood glucose, with resulting dehydration of the tissues and chemical imbalances that lead the patient to coma and sometimes to death. These effects clearly do not occur with either starvation or the ketogenic diet, in which glucose is restricted.*

Therefore, they thought I was crazy when I was saying the ketone would help, because they automatically thought of ketoacidosis and did not know any better.

Most people are ignorant about the difference between ketosis (i.e., ketone bodies in the urine while having normal blood glucose levels and not sick; as for example, Dr. freeman's patients on the ketogenic diet) and the deadly diabetic ketoacidosis (i.e., the combination of **both** ketone in urine and high blood glucose levels, not treated over a certain period of time with both ketosis and acidosis, **or** when sick and dehydrated with both ketosis and acidosis). They just did not understand what I was talking about. It was very frustrating.

I thought that I must not be the only parent with this kind of experience with their sick child, if I was right...so, I started asking parents of children with type 1 diabetes if they had experienced something similar (i.e., if they had gotten their child completely off insulin or been close to getting them off insulin following being sick with a high fever). I found about six parents who told me they had gone through similar experiences.

Next, I decided to try the forty-eight hours of fasting and the ketogenic diet along with my son. I used similar conditions as when he was hospitalized, using diet ginger ale during the fasting, and I was able to get him off insulin completely during the fasting. I observed that giving diet ginger ale during the fast was better than giving water from the tap because water would elevate the blood glucose for whatever unknown reason to me at that time. When you are on no insulin or practically no insulin, you see things that affect the body that are not covered up by insulin.

However, after the forty-eight hour fast and after starting the traditional ketogenic diet from Johns Hopkins, which is high in fat coming from dairy (with a lot of heavy cream), I had to put my son right back on insulin as it did not work with this type of diet/food. That was very disappointing. This particular diet (eating a lot of dairy) did not mimic at all the fasting results.

My son had a history of issues/allergies with dairy but I had hoped that since his body was being tricked into thinking it was starving, it might not affect him but I was wrong. It did not work.

I kept telling myself that I had just identified a way that did not work and I was getting closer to finding the right way. I kept thinking of this quote to give me motivation to keep going on, even though I was disappointed:

"I have not failed. I've just found
ten thousand ways that won't work."
~Thomas A. Edison

Indeed I did not fail. You will see later in chapter eight, after creating my own ketogenic diet, how different the results will be...

CHAPTER FIVE

Cancer Strikes, Not Once, But Twice

In 2010, I found out I had cancer after a period of great stress in my life, when I had been eating a lot of food from cans like soups and food from bags like corn chips with a lot of melted cheese, coffees with cream and a lot of low fat yogurts. I was diagnosed with breast cancer (i.e., invasive ductal adenocarcinoma). Without having any time to think after the shock of this news, within a week from diagnosis, I had a lumpectomy and three lymph nodes removed. My oncologist told me when the pathology came back that I had stage 2 cancer, which was more aggressive than previously thought. He said I had a strong grade 3 cancer...almost grade 4 out of 4 (er+/pr+, her2 negative), lymph nodes positive, and vascular invasion (in and out). I needed aggressive chemotherapy and radiation treatments or it would be in my vital organs and bones in no time.

I am a single mom. I work to support my kids and myself and to provide health insurance for us. I have a type I diabetic child to take care of who needs me and depends on me...this news was a shock. I had no time to be sick and to be off work and I needed to take care of my kids. People around me were crying and scared I would die...my mom, my sister, my nieces my friends, my kids...I had to keep strong for everyone.

I only cried a few tears one night when I was alone in bed, after my Oncologist had told me I needed an aggressive treatments, I had seen my daughter fighting the tears when the oncologist said it would be in my bones and vital organs in no time if I did not...I told the doctor that if I had to go, it would not be that way and I refused both chemotherapy and radiation. In the car, leaving the oncologist's office, my teenage daughter told me she supported my decision to refuse aggressive treatments. That meant so much to me.

I have watched two of my mom's sisters die from lung cancer, her other sister from breast cancer, and my dad's sister from breast cancer. On top of it, two good friends of mine recently died in their 40s from pancreas and lung cancer, suffering and leaving behind their young kids. I saw what chemotherapy and radiation did to them all and it sure did not cure them. I was there when they cried, when they lost their hair, when they could not breathe, when they had fluid on their lungs, when the white blood cell count was too low, when they were so sick from the treatments they could not get out of bed, when Elsa was in bed looking all skeletal, grabbing my arm and begging me to go tell her kids she loved them...

That just was not for me. I felt this stuff would kill me. I thought if I had to die, it would not be that way. But I was getting pressure from my oncologist to do at least radiation, so I went to the initial radiation oncologist visit. The doctor was extremely nice and I really liked her but her treatments just did not feel like they were right for me. I did not like it either when she told me that my lumpectomy area was very close to my lungs and my heart so they would have to measure and give me the radiation at an angle so I would only have very minimal chances of any lung/heart damage. I never went back and I cancelled the appointment they made for me to start radiation.

A family member told me to get the book *Knockout* [29] by Suzanne Somers. I ordered it right away and started to read it and other stuff to give myself a crash course on cancer. I loved this book. It felt right for me and my beliefs and it made a lot of sense to me. I was surprised to find out how intelligent Suzanne Somers really is and how smart to write her book with all these interviews with experts.

At the same time, I also became friends with Monique, who cured her stage 4 terminal breast cancer naturally. She was given six months to live, fourteen years ago. She was told she might last two years if she did chemotherapy and radiation. She refused both chemotherapy and radiation and said that the Doctor told her she was a very brave and smart woman at that time. She took tamoxifen (an estrogen blocker), changed her diet drastically based on Dr. Peter D'Adamo's book, *Eat Right 4 Your Type,* [30] she loaded up on vitamins and supplements, and cured her stage 4 terminal cancer naturally, even with metastases all over her back. She also gave me strength in my decision…the decision that felt right for me. After I told the Doctors I was refusing treatments, I felt like a ton of bricks were lifted from my shoulders. It felt great. I did not have to worry about the cancer treatments anymore and any stress/fears and other health complications that came along with them.

It made sense to me to refuse chemotherapy and radiation because they gave no guarantee that I would be cured and I saw the kind of death it brought to my relatives and my friends. The doctors were saying it would give me this-or-that percent chances that it would not come back again in the same spot for the radiation. I read about all the possible complications from chemo and radiation and I thought to myself that I had enough of the cancer problem without adding any additional health issues caused by chemotherapy and radiation. I did not feel like I wanted to lose my long hair, my eye lashes, eye brows, my teeth... I did not want to risk getting an even weaker immune system, another cancer from radiation, not feeling my arm, heart and lung problems, having a constant runny nose and sores in my nose because the hair did not grow back in my nose, having joint pains, etc...I also saw all the people I loved who died doing these conventional toxic treatments...it sure did not cure any of them. I wanted to live and I felt this would kill me and tear my body down...that was not what I needed to get healthier and that was not my preferred treatment. I did not want that.

After I made my decision, I just had to concentrate on getting back to being healthy from then on and take control of my own health. It made me happy to do things for myself to help me get better. Before, I did not like to cook but now all of a sudden, I was happy to cook to help myself with food. I started cooking and smiling.

I tried what my friend Monique told me she did for diet and for vitamins and supplements. She said for two to three years she did not eat dairy, pastas, bread, grains, rice, potatoes, sugar, and red meat, and she avoided processed foods (things in bags and boxes). She ate fresh white meat, fish, seafood, fresh veggies, eggs, olives, extra-virgin olive oil, coconut oil, nuts, green tea, and natural sugars if needed from fresh fruits, pure maple syrup, or pure honey.

I figured I was better off to model after someone who did something that actually worked, so I started to do what she told me right away. I also found my own little ways to eliminate stress from my life (breathing to oxygenate my body, relaxing, meditating, praying, listening to music, burning nice smelling candles, etc.). Thus, I started her diet and began taking the vitamins and the supplements. Within only a few days, I started feeling better and had more energy. The general fatigue that I had experienced when I had cancer was starting to leave me. Then, when my oncologist saw I was refusing chemotherapy and radiation, I was offered tamoxifen (hormone blockers), I accepted the prescription and started taking it.

Then I read some research about bromelain being good against cancer, so without thinking or researching this further, I started eating a lot of pineapple, which I thought contained bromelain. Unfortunately, about the same time I upped my fruit intake, I started to notice a lump that was growing in my breast in the same area where I had my surgery/lumpectomy. That was approximately four to five months after the lumpectomy. The cancer came back much bigger (some explain that by "angiogenesis").

I kept trying with the diet but the lump kept growing and was very hard and sticking out. I could see the color of my skin changing around the lump. My mom, my sister, and my best friend felt my lump in my breast and they were all serious and you could see they were scared for me.

Unfortunately, the diet that worked for Monique was not working for me. My cancer was too aggressive and kept growing. I had to figure out something else.

***

I kept trying to stay positive and I would listen to the song from Rascal Flatts called *Stand* about determination, courage and standing...I would read and read again things that I liked that motivated me like the following quotes:

"True strength is keeping everything together when everyone expects you to fall apart."~Unknown

***

Failure is only the opportunity to begin again more intelligently~ Henry Ford.

***

CHAPTER SIX

My Own Research

About two to three months after my lumpectomy I read about Coley's toxins and cancer remission. It was an article about injecting microbes to induce fever and achieving spontaneous cancer remissions. It piqued my curiosity and I started reading about Dr. William B. Coley, who was "inoculating his patients with an organism that caused erysipelas," in an attempt to cure them. Erysipelas is a bacterial infection, or a germ called "Streptococcus pyogenes" that induces high fever.

Just like what my son experienced, Dr. Coley's cancer patients would get sick with a high fever and some of the patients would be cured afterward. That was called instant remission. This was just too similar to the experience with my son to be a coincidence. I needed to learn more about this.

***

I started thinking about Dr. Go, who had told me, when my son was sick with the high fever that it was normal to have ketone when sick with fever and that it also happened to non-diabetics.

Therefore, I looked for medical research that would show that with high fever, you get high ketone in the urine. I came across the following articles that confirmed this:

"Exploring the clinical utility of blood ketone levels in the emergency department assessment of pediatric patients."[31] In the findings of this article, it is noted that there were higher levels of ketone in those with anorexia or in those exhibiting vomiting and fever.

From Wikipedia, I found out that conditions where the metabolism is increased, like fever, pregnancy and lactation, were also causes for ketosis and ketonuria.[32]

I also found additional information that again stated that vomiting, fever, and pregnancy could cause ketones but it also listed nutritional conditions such as starvation, fasting, high protein/low carbohydrate diets, and very low-calorie diets. This source also stated that high enough amounts of medium-chain triglycerides (MCTs) added to any diet could produce ketones.[33] [34]

Then I started looking into fasting and cancer to see if there were people who had cancer and who reported they were helped by fasting. I found information that stated the following:

"Fasting kills cancer for several reasons. It deprives the cancer cells of nutrition and, because it also deprives the body of nutrition, alkalizes the blood. Cancer can't grow in an alkaline environment. The pH of the blood is supposed to be slightly alkaline, but because the typical Western diet includes meat, sugar, caffeine, and other acid-forming foods, most people's blood is acidic, which is conducive to disease. It's not as much of a problem for a vegetarian who eats a grain-centered diet, but even whole-food desserts can acidify the blood. Salt or salty foods can counteract this, but I have a low tolerance for salt. Fasting would make my blood as alkaline as it was going to get. Another reason fasting kills cancer is that it unburdens the digestive system, which frees up a substantial portion of our energy (as much as 30%) ordinarily used for digestion, which can then be used for healing."[35]

I also found some anecdotes of people being cured of cancer using fasting. [36] [37]

Then I thought, when on a regular diet, if the main source of fuel for the body is

———————————

sugar/carbohydrates, then could sugar fuel the cancer since Monique told me not to eat any sugar other than natural sources? I then found various sources and Dr. Otto Warburg's research on Wikipedia that caught my attention:

"Cancer, above all other diseases, has countless secondary causes. But, even for cancer, there is only one prime cause. Summarized in a few words, the prime cause of cancer is the replacement of the respiration of oxygen in normal body cells by a fermentation of sugar." -- Dr. Otto H. Warburg."[38]

I found more information from Dr. Heise about Dr. Otto Warburg:

"Dr. Otto Warburg, Ph-D, a 1931 Nobel laureate in medicine, first discovered that cancer cells have a different energy metabolism compared to healthy cells. He found that malignant tumors frequently exhibit an increase in anaerobic ("without air") glycolysis -- an abnormal process whereby glucose is used as a primary fuel by cancer cells and which generates large amounts of lactic acid as a byproduct. In contrast, normal cells predominantly undergo aerobic ("with air") cellular metabolism. In cancer, the large increase in lactic acid generated by the cancer cells must be transported to the liver for metabolism and clearance. The lactic acid creates a lower, more acidic pH in cancerous tissues as well as overall physical fatigue from liver stress due to overworking to try to clear the lactic acid buildup.

Consequently, larger tumors tend to have a more acidic pH."[39]

The part about the cancer cells using glucose for fuel and producing large amount of lactic acids - which in turns makes a more acidic pH- got me curious as to what are sources of lactic acid.

From the website wisegeek, I found some information about lactic acid:

"Lactic acid, also known as milk acid or 2-hydroxypropanoic acid, is an acid that both is formed by the body. It also exists in some foods. In the body, lactic acid develops generally in conjunction with exercise. As for foods, lactic acid exists in certain milk products, like yogurt, as well as some processed foods like some breads and beers."[40] [41]

Some research also suggests that the blood pH in between cancer cells is more acidic and the more acidic pH promotes metastasis and more aggressive cancer.[42]

***

After looking at Dr. Coley's work with fever, it appears clear to me that Dr. Coley overlooked in his study the ketone bodies that are associated with fever and starvation. Ketone bodies are the by-product of the disease (while being sick and not eating). That is an important point because per a research paper titled "Cancer as a Metabolic Disease,"[43] cancer cells have trouble to process fat and ketones as a fuel source for energy but healthy cells thrive on fat and ketones.

Furthermore, to support my point on ketones and Coley, in looking at the best results for Coley's remission of cancer using toxins injections to induce fever, it appears that starvation keeps coming up:

"Since fever is a metabolic factor, the search for other factors should start by focusing on any other peculiarities that affected the metabolism of the patients who responded well to the toxins. One factor that comes up again and again when reading the narratives of the cancer patients who responded dramatically to Coley's toxins is starvation. In my view the incidence of undernourishment appears to be remarkably high in the anecdotal cases that are frequently touted as proof of the toxins. Indeed Coley's first patient had a sarcoma affecting his neck and tonsils. In fact it is said that the patient was in danger of dying from starvation. After several attempts, Coley succeeded in infecting him with a virulent strain of Streptococcus. He developed severe anorexia, vomiting and a high fever and his tumor began to shrink almost immediately. He went into

remission for eight years after just one attack of erysipelas."[44]

I looked at some of the historical data for Coley's patients who successfully went into remission to find out how long it took. For the patients who were the worst-case scenarios with very big tumors from what I could calculate, I found it took approximately two to five months of injections of toxins to produce remission. [45 46 47 48]

This made me think...if Coley's patients were kept with fever/injections for up to five months, it must have been unlikely that the patients were all starved (without any food) for this long of a period of time. What were these patients fed while having fever? Were they fed a diet that was low in carbohydrates so that it would not interfere with the ketones which are a symptom of disease? Were they fed a normal American diet with a lot of carbohydrates that could eliminate the ketones? Would the potency of the toxins even matter when it came to ketones, if the diet was very high in carbohydrates/glucose? Were they fed dairy that various research and studies link to cancer, type I diabetes, MS and other ailments? [49 50 51 52 53 54 55 56 57 58 59 60]

In trying to find information about what Coley's patients were fed during the time they were injected with the toxins and kept with fever, I stumbled upon the work of Dr. Max Gerson. I could not find any information for Coley's patients regarding diet, except starvation was involved in successful cases of remission.

Dr. Gerson had also used Coley's toxins, combined with his diet therapy, for some of his cancer patients who he was not able to help with diet alone. Contrary to Dr. Coley, Dr. Gerson had a very detailed diet therapy that he used in combination with Coley's toxins. [61] [62] [63]

In reviewing the Gerson diet, I noticed that it promoted fresh, unprocessed foods. It was free of major allergens (except for glucose coming from fruits/fructose) and it did not allow any dairy until after six to eight weeks from the start of the diet. Others following in Gerson's footsteps using

---

Coley's toxins have modified the Gerson diet and use cultured dairy from the start of the diet. They are unable to duplicate Gerson's fifty success stories published in his "best case series." [64]

Looking at others who use diet to treat cancer: Dr. Nicholas Gonzalez, in an interview with Dr. Mercola, talks about Dr. William Kelley's work and his own work treating cancer patients using different diets for different people and different cancers. Gonzalez also uses enzymes with his patients. [65] Digestive enzymes help with digestion, and systemic enzymes help throughout the body-immune functions, blood flow, blood circulation, etc.

***

Another important thing I came across is that some sources tell us that ketone alone is not enough to explain the success of the ketogenic diet. They say that ketone is only a marker that let us know that the body switched from burning glucose to burning fat for energy. This makes sense because even if ketone is achieved on the ketogenic diet, not all the patients that are in ketosis get successful results. It is also mentioned that when the ketogenic diet works, it is after an average period of nine days. [66] [67]

Furthermore, there is research that shows that cancer is linked to inflammation. [68] Dr. Eliaz also says in an article that there are more than one hundred types of autoimmune diseases, such as type I diabetes, lupus, MS, and Parkinson's, among others, and they are all characterized by "inflammatory immune responses".[69]

Thus, if all these diseases have inflammation in common, what can prevent inflammation? Well, in that same article from Dr. Eliaz, we read that removing allergens from the diet such as dairy, gluten and sugar can help, as well as exercise, supplements, detox and sleeping enough.

As well, COX-2 are enzymes linked to promoting inflammation. There are some easy, natural COX-2 inhibitors that we can use to reduce inflammation, such as resveratrol, modified citrus pectin (MCP), quercetin, curcumin, vitamin-C, Omega-3 fatty acids, and grape seed extracts, among others.[70 71 72 73 74 75 76 77]

———————————————

Let's look at a few examples of COX-2 inhibitors found in food sources. Resveratrol is found in peanuts and the skin of red grapes or in supplements. Quercetin is found in onions.
MCP is found in supplements or in the peel/zest of fresh lemon. Vitamin-C is found in supplements or in citrus fruits, such as lemon. A good source of omega-3 fatty acids is fresh fish, like salmon.

***

Glutathione is the major antioxidant in the body and it maintains the body pH to normal. Some foods and supplements boost glutathione and even HIV/AIDS patients benefit from glutathione- as well as other autoimmune disorders.[78] I find this interesting since coconut oil is said to have "antiviral" benefits. Could a ketogenic diet help HIV/AIDS patients as well?

***

Galectin-3 is also present in various cancers and linked to sugar and cancer spread. Research shows that modified citrus pectin (MCP) helps against that. [79]

There is a ketogenic diet for weight loss called the "Spanish Ketogenic Mediterranean Diet". This diet uses a lot of olive oil, which is said to be anti-inflammatory. However, this ketogenic diet, like most others, also has dairy in it, but a study shows that it is a healthy cardiovascular diet.[80]

A lot of critics of the ketogenic diet say it is bad for the kidneys and causes kidney stones but research actually shows otherwise. In fact, research shows it could possibly replace dialysis and reverse kidney failure, and supplements (listed on p. 99) can decrease chances for kidney stones. [81] [82] [83] As well, my version of the ketogenic diet does not restrict fluid intake (toxin free fluid) which also helps prevent kidney stones.

***

Per Wikipedia, pregnant women have higher acetone levels due to higher energy requirements. [84] Acetone is also linked to fever and is a symptom of disease just like fever is. I discussed earlier that the more fever, and vomiting, the more acetone and the more acetone, the more fever and it's a closed. Acetone is also one of the three ketone body sources.

I found an interesting story of a woman who was fighting cancer for months, using a healthy diet that appeared free of allergens. All of a sudden, the woman became pregnant and within a month she went into remission and became cancer free.[85] Didn't I just mention that pregnant women have higher levels of acetone and that acetone is a ketone body source?

Furthermore, FoxNews informed us about pregnancy hormone on April 20th, 2005. We were advised in an article that pregnancy hormone may prevent breast cancer. [86] Could it be that the HCG injections increase ketone levels in the urine, or could it be the HCG (low-carbohydrate) diet that goes with the injections increases ketone levels, or maybe both?

Research from the Institut de Physiologie in France shows that carbohydrates in the diet might be responsible for making cells cancerous. When the glucose/carbohydrates are removed, oxygen increases but when carbohydrates/glucose are brought back, there is fermentation of sugar without oxygen. The research suggests that cancer cells could be switched back to normal cells in the absence of glucose. [87] [88]

Dr. Burzynski, who has had a great deal of success with his cancer patients, as part of his treatment, his patients are put on supplements that are composed of amino acids, Curcumin, olive oil, piperine, and vitamin B2- among other things. These are all things in harmony with the research. Piperine is an alkaloid found in peppers and helps the body absorb nutrients.

Dr. Ann Wigmore who cured her own cancer, was using wheatgrass and wheatgrass contains almost all the amino acids.[89]

***

The carbohydrates the body needs can come from protein or fat. There is no known essential carbohydrate. Amino acids are the building blocks of proteins and proteins and fat are essential to life. [90]

***

"The food you eat can be either the safest

and most powerful form of medicine or the slowest form of poison."~ Dr. Ann Wigmore

***

Now let's do a recap of all the major points discussed in this chapter, so that all the links that became clear to me become clearer to my readers.

1- Per Dr. Otto Warburg, the primary cause of cancer is the fermentation of sugar without oxygen. Then cancer uses the sugar as a fuel and it generates lactic acids, which in turn creates a more acidic blood pH. The more acidic intercellular cancer cells blood pH is, the more aggressive the cancer.

2- We know the ketogenic diet switches the body to burning fat instead of glucose and mimics starvation-hence it gets rid of the sugar/glucose issue. Some research points to the ketogenic diet as to boosting glutathione and multiple research shows certain foods and supplements can also boost glutathione. Glutathione, per Dr. Nagasawa, is the major antioxidant in the body and is responsible for maintaining cellular redox homeostasis (meaning it maintains the pH at normal levels) as well as bringing oxygen to the cells.

3- Some foods are sources of lactic acids, such as dairy, bread, soy sauce, processed foods, etc.

4- Starvation (not eating any food) is linked to cancer remission, stopping seizures, decreasing blood glucose, decreasing insulin need, etc. Starvation produces ketones. Ketogenic diets mimic starvation.

5- Dairy is linked to cancer, type I diabetes, MS, and others diseases, and can be a source of lactic acid.

6- Most diseases have inflammation in common. Allergens in the diet are inflammatory and some foods and supplements are anti-inflammatory.

7- Ketogenic diets are actually good for the kidneys if you take the recommended supplements to lower the risks of kidney stones. There is even research that states that ketogenic diets can reverses diabetic kidney damage and could possibly replace dialysis.

8- The Spanish Mediterranean Ketogenic diet uses olive oil and a lot of fish, and is deemed via research to be good for the cardio-vascular system. It means no cholesterol issues as well.

9- Acetone is linked to fever. Pregnant women also have higher acetone levels.

10- Amino acids, proteins and fat are essential to life.

11- Research shows that cancer cells have trouble processing ketones and fat for energy to multiply, but healthy cells do not.

12- Research suggests that cancer cells can be switched back to healthy cells in the absence of glucose.

CHAPTER SEVEN

Creating my own ketogenic diet version and getting rid of cancer with diet

I decided to apply into my own ketogenic diet version, everything that I learned in my research. I wanted to live so it only made sense to put the most chances on my side and make my diet as full proof as I could. On January 3, 2011, I started my own ketogenic diet with a combination of **high fat** plus **high proteins** versus **low carbohydrates**. I used this combination in order to be able to remove the major allergens from my diet.

This way, I was able to remove dairy, glucose/fructose, soy, and grains. I removed red meat and dairy to avoid synthetic bovine growth hormone (rBGH), and I also wanted to avoid IGF-I from the cow's milk. I learned from Warburg and Heise that the primary cause of cancer is fermentation of sugar without oxygen and it causes a by-product of lactic acids- bringing down the pH. Therefore, I did not want to eat additional food sources of lactic acids either. I used healthy natural oils only that are linked to healthy cardio vascular system and many other benefits. I used only extra-virgin olive oil and organic extra-virgin coconut oil that have anti-cancer properties. [91] [92]

I started the diet without a fast. Therefore I knew that I would not have ketone in my urine within twenty-four hours, but it would take approximately fourty-eight hours before getting ketone.

I used non genetically modified organism (GMO) foods. That means no canola oil, no corn or corn oil, and no soy or soybean oil that contains GMOs. GMOs can become brand-new allergens, have lower nutrition, can become toxic and can cause cancer, as per Mr. Andrew Kimbrell (executive director at The Center for Food Safety in San Francisco, California), in the documentary film called *The Beautiful Truth*.[93]

In this same documentary, Dr. Russell Blaylock tells us that monosodium glutamate (MSG), often found in processed food, can interfere with brain function and is linked to several diseases such as diabetes, obesity, dementia, Parkinson's, cancer, and others.

The hidden terms for MSG are the following: monopotassium glutamate; glutamate; glutamic acid; gelatin; hydrolyzed vegetable protein; hydrolyzed plant protein; autolyzed plant protein; sodium caseinate; calcium caseinate; textured protein; yeast extract; yeast food or nutrient, and autolyzed yeast.

The documentary also informs us about the health dangers from mercury, fluoride, and aspartame. The importance of using detox to produce glutathione as transferase, to cleanse the blood, is also discussed.

I wanted to have the least amount of toxins possible going into my body, so I watched what I ate and drank and read every food label for the nutrition facts. That meant checking every single ingredient and putting things back on the grocery store shelves most of the time. It also meant shopping the perimeter of the grocery store and the organic section(s) for the fresh non-processed foods.

I bought a water filter to remove metals and chlorine. If I had a larger budget, I would have gotten a water filter that also removed fluoride and makes the water alkaline. However, I bought ion pods and manually made my water alkaline after it came out of my water filter. I tried to eat everything fresh and only non-processed foods as much as possible. There are some things that you cannot buy fresh, and that is okay as long as the ingredients do not list anything that is prohibited on my diet. For example, I like crab from Alaska and I cannot get it fresh living on the East Coast, so that is something I would buy frozen as long as it is not processed. I buy fresh wild salmon, chicken, and turkey and freeze it myself so I know there is no chemical added to it.

I avoided processed salt and used natural unprocessed sea salt instead.

I wanted to use healthy food like my friend Monique used to get rid of her stage 4 terminal cancer.

I used the ratios that Dr. Freeman used with his patients at Johns Hopkins because I figured he knew best, and I used the Dr. Atkins combo (high fat+high protein vs. low carbs) to produce the ketone-to be able to remove dairy- but I did not go by net carbs counting like the Atkins diet does. Instead, I counted total carbohydrates to remove the most carbohydrates and to produce the most ketone output to mimic what happens when you have a high fever. Therefore, I did not eat more than 20 to 30 grams of total carbohydrates per day and every time I ate or drank, I made sure I had no less than a 3:1 ratio (up to 5:1) of proteins and fat combined compared to the total carbohydrates.

I also used ketone urine testing strips to make sure that I always had a minimum measurement of moderate ketone but aiming for the maximum which is large on my product chart (40 to 160).

If I saw my ketone levels going down, I would eat fat in the form of raw coconut oil to bring my ketone levels back up. You can't be afraid to eat healthy fat on my diet. Healthy fat is cancer's enemy. Remember, in my research section, I wrote that cancer cells have trouble processing fat for energy to multiply, but healthy cells do not and thrive on fat.

On January 7, 2011, I had a scheduled appointment with my Oncologist. He felt my lump and told me that it was a recurrence- it was hard, sticking out, consistent with cancer, and it was coming back in the same area as the lumpectomy because I had refused radiation. It was about the size of a small egg at that time (the Surgeon later told me that the oncologist wrote in my report that it was approximately a 2cm tumor). The oncologist said he was treating this very seriously and tried to rush me to the surgeon's office. The surgeon's office actually called me for an appointment while I was still in the parking lot of the oncologist's office.

I did not want to be rushed into surgery this time. I wanted to give my diet some time to work, as I knew I was just starting to get ketone in my urine, and was starting to switch my body fuel to fat, and I had just depleted the sugar reserves in my body. So, I told the surgeon's office I could not go until January 14th.

I concentrated on my diet, eating foods and spices with anti-cancer properties. I used foods and supplements to boost glutathione. I used sources of iron, iodine, amino acids, various nutrients, and antioxidants.

I kept telling myself one of my favourite quotes:

"If anything is worth doing, do it with all your heart." –Buddha

I also kept telling myself what my sister told me to tell myself: my cells regenerate themselves in the Divine order. I tried to avoid any stress and got enough sleep making sure I slept in a darkened room. I used 3mg of melatonin supplement before going to sleep.

Here are some examples of things I would eat: black olives, olive oil mayonnaise, extra-virgin olive oil, organic coconut oil, eggs (poached, fried, omelettes with a little water to fluff them, hard-boiled), chicken, turkey, all fish and seafood (especially salmon, haddock, shrimps and sardines with fresh lemon juice), organic seaweeds from Maine, mixed nuts, peanuts (which have resveratrol) and almonds. I would drink boiled water with lemon, green tea with either lemon or mint to alkalize, mineral water, and the anti-inflammatory lemonade (recipe provided in Chapter 11). I would get my few carbs from fresh cruciferous and fresh low-carbs veggies such as Brussels sprouts, bok choy, spinach, asparagus, cauliflower, broccoli, watercress, and kale.

To spice up my food, I used the following that have direct or indirect cancer-fighting properties: lemon, cayenne pepper, parsley, turmeric/curcumin, garlic and garlic powder, cumin, onions (has quercetin), watercress, cilantro (also called coriander), basil, healthy unprocessed sea salt with iodine and minerals, black pepper and all sorts of peppers (they contain piperine), rosemary, paprika, saffron, thyme, fennel, ginger, cardamom, and cinnamon. I would use at least a minimum of three of these for every meal I would eat.

I also took my non-synthetic multi-vitamins with enzymes, minerals, and herbs as advised by my friend Monique and all my anti-cancer supplements (listed in Chapter 10). After reading the life story of Ann Wigmore, I started drinking wheatgrass to alkalize my body and to get all of the essential amino acids. I was also getting amino acids in poultry, nuts, eggs and fish.

My goal was to get rid of as many free radicals, toxins, and allergens in my body as possible; to boost my immune system; to get ketones to starve my cancer; and try to turn my cancer cells back into healthy cells.

On January 10 or 11 (approximately seven days after beginning my diet), I started to feel my lump decrease little by little and it did not feel as hard as it did before. At the same time as the cancer started shrinking, I started to experience aches and pains and suction-like feelings. I could feel a trace of the pain from where the lump was, going all around my left breast and towards my arm. I also felt pain where my lump was, going straight through my back. That scared me a little at first, but a friend told me it might be a sign my immune system was kicking in and that reassured me. I later found documentation on tumor pain that explains pain during tumor healing is a common occurrence. [94] [95]

When I first felt the lump shrink, I thought maybe it was just my imagination- I wanted it to go away so badly that perhaps it was just in my mind. But each day I kept feeling my breast and it kept going down in size. I was feeling great on my diet and I was so happy to feel my lump shrinking so quickly. It was exciting. I was smiling all the time.

By January 14, when I went to see the surgeon, my lump was down to approximately a tiny bit smaller than the size of a kidney bean. The surgeon did a sonogram and a needle biopsy and said it was not cancer from looking at the sonogram. I asked if she could tell on the sonogram if it was dead cancer cells, but she said it was too hard to tell and she could only say if it was or was not cancer. The biopsy also came back negative and a few days later, the lump was completely gone (approximately two weeks after I started my diet). The surgeon said that cancer does not shrink and seemed to think that the oncologist might have made a mistake. The oncologist wrote the size of my tumor as approximately 2 cm in his referral to the surgeon and I had almost nothing left. I told the surgeon that I did not doubt my oncologist at all.

The oncologist's office still wanted me to go for a mammogram after the negative results and called me to schedule a mammogram. They seemed to have trouble believing this tumor was gone. I refused the mammogram.

I stayed on my strict ketogenic diet for two months to be on the safe side, even though my lump was gone after two weeks. I based my reasoning on Dr. Coley's work- I looked for how long he kept his worst-case scenario patients with fever/ketones and found out that it was two to five months before getting them in remission. That was the ones who had huge tumors, who were in really bad shape and in danger of dying. Others in less dire need were in remission faster than that.

Since then, I've regained my energy. I am fine and lead a normal life. I have stopped taking tamoxifen since it did not prevent me from getting a recurrence, and I am not on any prescription medication. My oncologist put in my medical file that I am in complete remission. Last time I saw my oncologist (January 2012), all my blood test results were in normal range and so were my liver and kidney functions.

I did not do any calorie restriction while on my diet and I did not restrict liquid intake either. I had as much food as I needed and I drank as much as I needed. I just made sure every time I put something in my mouth to drink or eat, it had either no total carbs in it or had at least a minimum 3:1 ratio ([Protein+Fat]: [Total Carbs]) up to a 5:1 ratio. My weight stayed stable, my skin became soft and my energy level went back up.

As I said, I stayed on my own ketogenic version-THE CANTIN KETOGENIC DIET- for two months to get rid of my cancer. I now use my cancer preventive diet, which is basically the same thing except I do not keep the strict ketogenic ratio anymore and I now eat more carbohydrates from my permitted list of foods. I still try my best to stay away from what is on the prohibited list. I also added some additional foods, like sweet potatoes, quinoa and some fruits but mostly berries- fresh fruits that contain the most antioxidants and the least sugar.
I am still avoiding red meat, bread, pastas, grains, sugar, dairy, soy, and processed food as much as I can, but I have upped my intake of carbohydrates coming from fresh veggies.

I try my best to balance my hormones naturally to boost my anti-carcinogenic hormones with food, vitamins, and supplements. I did the 2/16 and twenty-four hour hormonal urine tests and the results were either in normal range or almost in normal range. I used a lot of info from the book *Knockout*"⁹⁶ and the interview with Dr. Wright to balance my hormones, using tools like a low carbohydrate/sugar diet, iodine from seaweeds, green leafy veggies, cruciferous veggies at least three times a week, sam-e supplement, vitamin B12, folic acid, betaine, exercise, and so on.

Every six months, I go back on my ketogenic diet for a minimum of fifteen to twenty days in order to prevent recurrence. My reasoning for the length was based on my cancer being gone after about fifteen days, and on Dr. Geyelin that said that the best period of time of fast for curing his epileptic patients was twenty days (this observation with his patients matches with my experience).

Just some thoughts that motivated me…

***

He is able who thinks he is
able.~Buddha
***

If something is worth doing, do it with all
your heart~Buddha

***

Nothing in life is to be feared, it is only to
be understood. Now is the time to
understand more, so that we may
fear less. ~ Marie Curie

***

CHAPTER EIGHT

My Son, Type I Diabetes, and My Own Ketogenic Diet Version

Back to my son and type I diabetes. So now, armed with the knowledge of a healthy, allergen-free ketogenic diet without dairy, soy, etc…

In August 2011, I tested my diet on my son. Without doing a fast first (since I already knew that fasting gets him completely off insulin), I put my son on my own version of the ketogenic diet-the same diet I used to make my tumor disappear. Unlike the traditional ketogenic diet, on my own version of the ketogenic diet, my son was able to eat without taking any insulin bolus for the food and without needing any insulin correction since the blood glucose (BG) was staying leveled in the 100s.

From the time he started having ketones, he needed only a basal insulin rate and it kept decreasing with time.

I also observed that drinking alkaline water (tap water that went through a water filter to remove the metals and chlorine, and then alkalized in an ion pod) would make the blood glucose drop. I find this very interesting because in the book *The Ketogenic Diet,* [97] it says that administering excess water can provoke seizures and mentions the need to limit fluids on the traditional ketogenic diet. It also discusses the misconceptions about water affecting sodium levels and diluting the urine ketones, which does not affect the blood and brain ketone levels.

What about the scientific research about the toxic effects of chlorine and fluoride in the water and the links found to Alzheimer's disease (AD) and the effects it has on the brain? [98] [99] [100] [101] [102] [103]

Furthermore, what about fluoride being identified as weakening the immune system; causing allergic-type reactions; causing birth defects; causing genetic damage; and being likely to aggravate kidney disease, diabetes and hypothyroidism?[104]

I did not restrict my own fluid intake while on the ketogenic diet and I did not restrict my son's fluid intake either. However, I controlled the kind of fluid that went into my body and his body. I used a water filter that I bought for around forty-nine dollars that removes or decreases lead,

---

mercury, benzene, asbestos, pesticides, herbicides, chlorine, chlorination by-products, pharmaceuticals, and microbial cysts. Then I put the filtered water into an ion pod for three minutes to make the water more alkaline.

I observed that drinking this filtered and alkalized water dropped my son's blood glucose after drinking only one or two cups.

I want to point out here that earlier when I described our attempt at fasting, the water from the tap (which was not filtered and not alkaline) was raising my son's blood glucose. During the fast, I switched back to using diet ginger ale instead of tap water to get him off insulin completely during the fast (just like when he was hospitalized).

My son is on an insulin pump. Right away when he started having ketones in his urine on my ketogenic diet version, the basal rate had to be dropped constantly so I had to decrease the basal rate down gradually until it was 0.5 unit per hour of short acting insulin (I added a basal pattern on his pump to drop the basal rate). He was eating without needing insulin bolus for the food and without needing insulin bolus for correction as the blood glucose was staying stable. After a week on the diet, he was almost completely off insulin with only a minimal basal rate. I thought this was an amazing result after such a short period of time. However, he started eating carbohydrates again and the ketone levels dropped. He asked/begged for a break because it was too hard for him to follow this restrictive diet.

Unfortunately, he does not have the discipline that I have. He had been a diabetic for over thirteen years at this point (since he was two) and I had no clue how long it would take on my diet to keep him on this diet for his body to possibly start making beta cells again, as suggested in the research paper titled "Research shows promise in reversing Type 1 diabetes". [105]

In essence, the findings of this research state: "The findings contradict an essential paradigm of diabetes therapy — that once the insulin-secreting beta cells of the pancreas have been destroyed, they are gone forever. Because of that belief, most research today focuses on using vaccines to prevent the cells' destruction in the first place, or on using beta cell transplants to replace the destroyed cells. The new findings, however, hint that even in patients with long-standing diabetes, the body retains the potential to restore pancreas function if clinicians can only block the parts of the immune system that are killing the beta cells. "

I just know that I have now found the way to mimic fasting in my son's body using my own version of the ketogenic diet. Very importantly, unlike the Allen starvation treatment, because my diet mimics fasting, there is no need for calorie restriction at all. My son could eat as much as he wanted and the blood glucose would stay in the 100s and would go back down on its own-right from the start. It was amazing to see and exciting.

My son's behavior and mood were also so improved during that week and it was like he was a different person. His A1C test results also dropped even if it was just a week.

***

It appears this might be stopping the autoimmune reaction that kills the beta cells. Remember, when I described earlier that my son was hospitalized and sick, it was like he was cured for three days after the fever and vomiting with large ketone. This just needs to be proven and if it is, that means that my ketogenic diet version stops the autoimmune reaction that kills the beta cells and could allow the restoration of pancreas functions that research hint is possible. This research also seems to be in harmony with what happened to my son in real life, so I have faith this will be the case.

If it is proven to be so, it means that my ketogenic diet version is the natural cure for type I diabetes and it is available right now with no harm needed. This is just the beginning…

***

IMPORTANT NOTES:

These results for my son now give some hope for type I diabetics who have developed antibodies to insulin and for those who experience "extreme insulin resistance"- the ones who are on hundreds of units of insulin per day and still cannot lower their blood glucose. They now have an alternative with my ketogenic diet.

My diet is the only ketogenic diet version, as far as I know, that is free of dairy, major allergens, and toxins. Therefore, it is very important to note that all the tests and published researches with the ketogenic diets were most likely done with dairy and other allergens allowed in the diets. This might have affected the results of these studies. It might also make a difference for the epileptic patients whom the traditional diet did not work for.

There is plenty of research that shows that dairy can be bad for the health of cancer patients, MS patients, epileptic patients, diabetic patients, and others. If dairy allergies or beef protein allergies or any other food allergies or antibodies can cause such a reaction inside our bodies, we should stay away from such foods to be able to mimic fasting while on a ketogenic diet. I have demonstrated with my son's case and with my own case the positive results on the outcome.

***

Let me end this chapter with the wise
words I was told by a lady who I admire greatly:

"Results are undisputable. I never argue with
results."~ Charlotte Gerson

THE CANTIN KETOGENIC DIET

CHAPTER NINE

Coming up with a Mathematical Formula to Bring in Logic

For both cancer and type I diabetes, I decided to come up with a mathematical formula to show my point logically. Due to the similarities in conditions with what happened to my son when he was sick with high fever (starvation) then getting completely off insulin for three full days and for Dr. Coley's patients who were sick with high fever (starvation) and sometimes getting cancer remission, I came up with a mathematical formula to show how to produce remission without the fever and without starving, by using ketones and a ketogenic diet instead.

I started with Dr. Warburg's scientific research because he won the Nobel Prize for his cancer research. Then, I tried to see if I could find a link between Dr. Warburg's scientific research (which showed that glucose fuels cancer) and Dr. Coley's work and his practical real-life experience with curing patients and sometimes producing cancer remission - something that removes the fermentation of sugar (or glucose) then equals remission (sometimes) for both Dr. Coley's cancer patients and for my son with type I diabetes. For my son, it eliminated the need for insulin or decreased it to nothing, if you prefer.

Therefore:

X – GLUCOSE = REMISSION (SOMETIMES)

The X variable with Coley's patients can either be the DISEASE (starvation) caused by the toxins OR the FEVER OR BOTH.

Thus:

DISEASE (starvation) and/or FEVER (starvation) – GLUCOSE = REMISSION (sometimes)

We have evidence, as discussed previously with supporting references for the following: both the DISEASE (starvation) and FEVER (starvation) are associated to KETONE bodies; starvation produces ketones and the ketogenic diet, which mimics fasting/starvation, also produces ketones.

We also discussed that ACETONE (which is one of the ketone bodies) and FEVER are symptoms of illness/disease (starvation) that are both linked together and can create a closed loop (i.e., like a vicious circle, the more acetone, the more fever and vomiting, and the more fever, the more acetone).[106] As well, loss of appetite usually accompanies fever. [107]

This means that acetone is linked to both disease (starvation) and fever. Acetone is also linked to subtracting the glucose in the body because it is one of the three ketone body sources (along with acetoacetate and beta-hydroxybutyrate). The presence of ketones indicates that the body is burning fat for energy instead of glucose.

In other words, we can say:

DISEASE (starvation) = KETONE body sources

FEVER (disease and starvation)=
ACETONE(disease and starvation)

ACETONE=ketone body source

Ketogenic diet or starvation= ketone body sources

Then we can also replace the "DISEASE (starvation)" by the KETONES in the equation, and the FEVER by ACETONE:

KETONE body sources (starvation) and/or ACETONE – GLUCOSE = REMISSION (sometimes)

Ketone body sources can also be replaced in the formula by ketogenic diet.

KETOGENIC DIET (which mimics starvation) and/or ACETONE – GLUCOSE = REMISSION (sometimes)

This formula can now be applied to both type I diabetes and cancer and it possibly can be applied to other ailments as well.

However, we still are left with the word "SOMETIMES" in my formula to be explained logically. Why is it that sometimes Coley's patients would go into remission and sometimes they would not? Let's look at some important points to try to make sense of this...

A) In Coley's case studies, I read that sometimes the toxin injection was killing the patients, possibly due to the potency of the toxins. What if it was not potent enough? You might not have as many ketones or you might not have any ketones.

B) With my son's case study with type I diabetes, we show that the allergen(s) also have to be considered. It shows that in his body, the traditional ketogenic diet did not mimic fasting (starvation), as he was able to be completely off insulin during fasting (starvation) and had to be put back on insulin when starting the traditional ketogenic diet, which is high in dairy (even if he had the desired ketone output). However, as I have explained, when put on my own modified ketogenic diet without the major allergens (including no dairy) and with the least toxins, he was able to gradually decrease the insulin to nothing and eat a normal daily caloric intake because this allergen-free ketogenic diet mimics fasting (starvation) in his body. Just eating the types of food on my ketogenic diet decreases the insulin need in his body even without having ketone (the traditional ketogenic diet does not do that). This is an indication that my allergen-free ketogenic diet works in harmony with the ketone for his body and that allergens affect blood glucose.

C) In Coley's case studies: "One factor that comes up again and again when reading the narratives of the cancer patients who responded dramatically to Coley's toxins is starvation. Indeed Coley's first patient had a sarcoma affecting his neck and tonsils. In fact it is said that the patient was in danger of dying from starvation. After several attempts, Coley succeeded in infecting him with a virulent strain of Streptococcus. He developed severe anorexia, vomiting, and a high fever, and his tumor began to shrink almost immediately." [108]

D) In my own cancer case study, my cancer tumor recurrence was completely gone in approximately two weeks on my own diet. I aimed for maximum ketones just like those produced by a high fever. I tried to avoid anything that could affect my body negatively to free up my immune system. Just like when you fast and do not eat at all so that nothing can impact on the body negatively coming from food.

E) Max Gerson also experimented with Coley's toxins combined with the Gerson diet for some of his patients when the diet alone was not enough or did not produce remission of cancer. Gerson's diet is also free of major allergens. He was using an allergen-free diet combined with the toxins injections that caused a disease and produced fever and ketones. Ketones and fever are symptoms of the disease. It is unknown however, the precise ratio of fruits/fructose in the diet compared to the low-carbohydrate veggies that the patients were ingesting and the urine ketone levels. That could possibly affect results. Gerson also did not allow any dairy in the diet until six to eight weeks after the start of the diet. In looking at Coley's case studies and at my own, some patients would have enough time to already go into remission after six to eight weeks. However, in Coley's case studies for the worst-case-scenario patients, it took about two to five months to go into remission. If they had an allergy to the diet that could have possibly affected the blood glucose negatively, and affected the results of Gerson's studies.

F) Gerson's successors, who use Coley's toxins along with a modified version of Gerson's diet, use cultured dairy in the diet from the beginning. They are unable to consistently duplicate Gerson's good results (fifty cases), which were published in Gerson's monograph before his death.

G) In the Allen (starvation) treatment, the case studies for Type I diabetes show that patients were fed dairy, grains and fruits (fructose). They could not eat a diet with a normal daily caloric intake; they had to be kept in starvation and eat almost nothing in order to stay alive before insulin was discovered. If they ate too much, they had to go back on a fast (starvation) until the blood glucose (BG) went back down to normal before they could start to eat again. This was not the case for my son on my allergens-free (including dairy free) ketogenic diet, on which he can eat as much as he wants and the blood glucose will remain in normal range. This is an indication the Allen treatment did not mimic fasting and that my diet mimics fasting/starvation. This is also an indication that the types of foods we eat matters and can make a big difference.

H) Dr. Nicholas Gonzalez uses the Atkins diet with some of his cancer patients but it does not work for all. It appears to be due to different allergens in the diet, affecting different people differently. Here is an important quote from Dr. Gonzalez:

"Kelley differed from some of the alternative practitioners who were treating cancer, like Gerson, who preceded Kelley, who had one diet for everybody. One of Kelley's genius innovations which you know about, because I

know you're big on metabolic typing, is that different people need different diets. When I met Kelley, he had ten basic diets that he used that ranged from pure vegetarian, nuts and seeds, and raw food to red meat three times a day, like an Atkins diet. He had ten basic diets and ninety variations that were all on his computer. His attitude was that different people need different types of cancer treatment. His program and our program today have three basic components: individualized diets, individualized supplement programs with large doses of enzymes, and the third component is detoxification routine. "[109]

I) In the book *Breahthrough*, there is a quote that indicates that the diet used before the discovery of insulin was not in harmony with ketone for Type I diabetics, as it did not mimic fasting.

"Diet made with cream, eggs, bran rusks, vegetables boiled three times to purge them of carbohydrates. No desserts or bread ever... The less food, the more life... To starve is to survive". [110]

They were not keeping them alive for more than eighteen months with 400 calories per/day on that diet (if they survived the diet). Diet down from 2000 calories per day to 400 calories per day for Elizabeth Hugues in the book (she was twelve years old). They were fed allergens such as dairy (i.e., cream) and grains (i.e., bran).

Therefore, it appears from the case studies and from my own experience as well as my son's, that the "sometimes" referring to remission of cancer and type I diabetes, when it comes to ketogenic diets OR fever, can be explained depending on the foods in the diet. Here are the possible outcomes per the studies and my experiences:

1. You get positive results with: fasting/starvation as long as there are no allergens or toxins in the fluid intake OR with a ketogenic diet that is free of allergens/toxins and mimics fasting.

2. You get negative results with a diet that does not mimic fasting.-a diet with allergens (that affect blood glucose) and toxins AND/OR a diet with enough glucose to interfere with the ketone levels.

Now, let's bring back my mathematical formula and add the last findings:

KETONE body sources (starvation or ketogenic diet) and/or ACETONE – GLUCOSE = REMISSION (when there is fasting/starvation with fluid intake free of allergen/toxins OR with a ketogenic diet that is allergens/toxins free that mimics fasting).

***

IMPORTANT NOTE: This now links my ketogenic diet to immunotherapy.

CHAPTER TEN:

THE CANTIN KETOGENIC DIET: How to Do the Diet

Again, a reminder that this diet should only be done under medical supervision.

I modified the traditional ketogenic diet-using the books from Dr. John M. Freeman & from Dr. Robert C. Atkins, as previously referenced.

A ketogenic diet is a diet that is supposed to mimic fasting and switches our body to burning fat for energy instead of glucose. I used Atkins combination of **[Fat + Protein]:[carbs]** intake to be able to produce the ketone in a way that allowed me to remove major allergens from the diet such as dairy, soy, grains, etc. This is different than the traditional ketogenic diet.

The traditional ketogenic diet uses the **[Fat]:[protein + carbs]** combination to produce ketone and uses a lot of dairy & various allergens, unless the patient comes in already advising the medical staff that there is a known allergy. With the traditional ketogenic diet, protein is also limited and should not be more than approximately 1 gram per kilogram of weight (this is not the case for my ketogenic diet, protein is not limited). The Atkins diet also uses a lot of dairy and various allergens so this is why I created my own version of the diet, removing most allergens and toxins to get the best possible outcome. Any additional known allergens should also be removed from the diet. I also used the ratios from Dr. John M. Freeman –a minimum of 3:1 ratio but aiming for a 4 to 5:1 ratio. I go by total carbs to eliminate the most carbs unlike the Atkins diet, which goes by net carb counting. I wanted to produce elevated ketone levels similar to ketone levels that are produced when a person is sick with a high fever. I ate no more than 20–30 grams of carbohydrates per day to achieve that (under 20 grams for a non-vegan and up to 30 grams for a vegan).

I removed: dairy, red meat, soy, wheat, grains, and fructose (except for a few berries) from my diet and most of my fat intake was from mainly healthy fat sources such as extra-virgin olive oil and pure coconut oil, due to their health benefits for the cardio-vascular system, cholesterol, anti-cancer properties, and benefits for other ailments. [111] [112]

PROHIBITED FOOD LIST:

Alcohol
Corn
Canola
Chips
Dairy (butter, milk, cream, cheese, yogurts, whey,
        casein, curd, etc.)
Fruits (except for a few blueberries, blackberries,
        and raspberries after the cancer is gone)
Genetically modified organism (GMO) food
Grains
Processed foods
Red meat
Rice
Salt that is processed
Soy
Sugar/fructose
Vegetable oils (including canola oil)
Water (from tap without a filter to remove
        chlorine, metals, and other toxins)
Wheat

***IMPORTANT: any foods that are known allergens or are known to cause any negative reactions in the body of the person doing this diet should be added to this prohibited list.

 Basically, I tried to eat mostly fresh organic foods with as little as possible carbohydrates/sugar, no processed food with unknown ingredients, no major allergens, and the least possible toxins.

PERMITTED FOOD LIST:

Almonds

Almond milk, unsweetened

Almond flour

Cacao butter, Organic/raw

Chicken

Chicken broth or vegetable broth, organic and low
   sodium

Coconut oil, extra virgin/ organic

Coconut milk, unsweetened

Eggs, organic (poached, fried, omelets, hard-
      boiled)

Fish (especially salmon, haddock, and sardines)

Green tea

Healthy unprocessed sea salt

Herbs (cilantro/coriander, parsley)

Lemon

Lime

Mayonnaise

Medium-chain triglycerides (MCT) oil

Mineral water

Olives and olive oil (extra-virgin)

Nuts

Peanuts and organic natural peanut butter

Protein powder (ketogenic, plant-based without
      allergens made with: pea protein, cranberry
      protein, hemp protein, and Medium Chain
      Triglycerides MCT)

Salt (unprocessed natural sea salt)

Seafood

Seaweeds, organic (kelp, dulse, spirulina, etc.)

Spices (turmeric/curcumin, ginger, garlic, peppers, etc.)

Stevia

Turkey

Vegetables (especially low-carbs and cruciferous/brassica)

Water from the tap (filtered to remove chlorine, metals, and other toxins or at least boiled). Optionally alkalized through a water purification system that removes fluoride or ion pods to alkalize.

***

I drank boiled water with lemon, mineral water, filtered/alkaline water, anti-inflammatory lemonade (recipe provided in Chapter 11), or decaffeinated green tea with lemon or mint.

I ate my few carbohydrates from fresh cruciferous and other low-carb vegetables like Brussels sprouts, bok choy, spinach, asparagus, cauliflower, broccoli, watercress, kale, and mixed salad, etc.

I used the following to spice up my food (things that are anti- cancer directly or indirectly by boosting the immune system): lemon, cayenne pepper, parsley, mint, turmeric/curcumin, garlic and garlic salt, cumin, onions, olives, watercress, cilantro (also called coriander), basil, unprocessed sea salt with iodine and minerals, black pepper, peppers, rosemary, paprika, saffron, thyme, fennel, ginger, cardamom, and cinnamon.

I used at least a minimum of three of these for every meal I ate.

I also drank two ounces of aloe vera juice, two to three times per day. I picked a particular organic brand because it had less than one gram of total carbs per two ounces. I took wheatgrass daily because it is alkaline and for its content of amino acids. Dr. Burzynski's supplements are also loaded with amino acids.

Instead of doing coffee enemas like some choose to do, I chose to detoxify my body in a different way. I used modified citrus pectin (MCP) as a gentle detox along with other natural foods and supplements. I made sure I had fresh lemon in warm water first thing in the morning, during the day, and before bed. I used turmeric/curcumin and fresh lemon for the liver. I used fresh parsley for the kidneys. I used cilantro/coriander and seaweeds to eliminate toxins. I also used a SAM-e supplement to boost glutathione transferase.

The organic raw seaweeds from Maine, which I would eat for snacks, also gave me iron and iodine. Iron is linked to oxygen and iodine boosts anti-carcinogenic estrogen hormones.

Some supplements I took just during the initial diet and some I still take daily: the supplement from nurse Renee Caisse (for three months), an organic multivitamins (with herbs, including spirulina, Chinese skullcap, minerals, and enzymes), another organic multi-vitamin (with systemic and digestive enzymes, raw food extract, CoQ10, iodine, herbs, and more), green tea, NAC, spirulina, chlorella, kelp, astragalus, reishi mushroom, astaxanthin, quercetin, and DIM.

Some COX-2 inhibitors (anti-inflammatories) that I took included turmeric/curcumin, melatonin (I also slept in a very dark room to boost melatonin), modified citrus pectin (MCP), vitamin C, quercetin, and resveratrol.

***

NOTE FOR VEGANS:

You can also do this diet if you are vegan using the list of permitted food and the following:

Almond flour (without any added ingredients) or other nut flours like hazelnut, pecan or walnut flour with at least a 3:1 ketogenic ratio for the FAT+Proteins compared to total carbohydrates.

Almond butter and peanut butter.

Vegetables with a lot of protein such as spinach, artichokes, collards, and others on the permitted list.

Plant protein powder that is allergen-free and ketogenic. It is a raw protein that is plant-based, gluten-free, sugar-free, dairy-free, hypo-allergenic, non-GMO, fortified with coconut (MCT) oil, AND made with pea protein, cranberry protein, hemp protein, and medium chain triglycerides-with a 18:1 ketogenic ratio (17 gr. of protein, 1.2 gr. of fat, and only 1 gr. of total carb). Use protein shakes if you are still hungry between meals or at night (this particular kind).

Vegan mayonnaise recipes made (for example) with cashews or almonds, olive oil, apple cider vinegar, garlic, lemon juice, and healthy sea salt.

The healthy fats listed on the permitted list and MCT oil.

DAY	Menu Example for Vegans
Breakfast	At least two scoops of the plant protein powder (36.4 grams of protein+fat and 2 grams of total carbs); sliced fresh avocado (3 grams total carbs). 1 Cup almond milk=1 gram of total carbs.
Morning Snack	Almonds (1/4 cup=5 grams total carbs) or seeds
Lunch	At least two scoops of the plant protein powder (36.4 grams protein+fat; 2 grams total carbs); fresh spinach salad (2 cups = 2 grams total carbs); raw cacao butter=zero carbs
Afternoon Snack	Seaweeds (3 grams total carbs)
Dinner	At least 2 scoops of the plant protein powder (36.4 grams of protein+fat and 2 grams of total carbs); asparagus (1/2 cup=2 total carbs); green salad (2 cups=2 grams total carbs); black olives 2 grams total carbs/10 olives

THE CANTIN KETOGENIC DIET
SOME OF THE MAJOR POINTS FOR MY DIET

Number 1-

This diet should be done under medical supervision. The key for success for my diet, per my experience and my son's, is that you need all three of the following for it to work (ketone alone will not work). You need:

A) ketone

B) to remove allergens: use the Cantin Ketogenic diet to remove the major allergens/toxins (dairy, soy, wheat/grains, fructose, rBGH, GMO, etc.) and remove any other known allergens that may be present in the diet or in the environment.
C) to remove toxins/stress (for examples: use a water filter to remove chlorine and metals and/or boil water. You can also use an ion pod to alkalize the water or use some other system. For stress, use breathing techniques, candles, aroma-therapy, etc.

Number 2-

I bought urinalysis testing strips to check my urine ketone levels. My goal was to keep the ketone at least moderate but I aimed for the maximum. Ketone is the key to starve the cancer. It makes you eliminate the acid in your body through the urine (therefore do not bother checking urine pH as it will be acidic). The presence of ketone indicates that you have now switched your body to burning fat as its source of energy instead of burning glucose. It means you have depleted the sugar reserves in your body. At all times, I was trying to achieve at least moderate ketone or more (to mimic being sick with a high fever). I was trying to stay away from only having "trace" ketone because that would mean that I was on the fence between having ketone and losing ketone and reverting back to using glucose for my body energy source. Ketogenic diets mimics fasting and put your immune system into combat mode for you. After seven to 10 days on this diet, the body's homeostasis properties kick in, bringing the body into equilibrium and pH to close to normal.

Number 3-

Every time I would eat or drink, I kept a ratio of at least 3:1 up to 5:1 for the combination of **[Fat + Protein]:[carbs]** (e.i., FAT + PROTEIN must be at least three to five times the amount of total carbs). This is to keep enough ketone in the urine. If you want to get more ketone, you just decrease the amount of carb intake and up the fat and protein intake. My daily total carb intake was up to 20gr for non-vegan and up to 30 grams of total carbs per day for vegan. Again this is different than the traditional ketogenic diet that uses **[Fat]:[protein + carbs]** combination and restricts protein.

To lose weight on this diet, you just need to decrease the amount of daily calories to a lower amount than what your body needs to maintain its weight. To gain weight, then you just make sure you take in more daily calories than what you need to maintain weight.

You can adjust the daily calorie intake to your needs as long as you keep having ketones to starve the cancer and you stay away from the major allergens. Use urinalysis strips to test the urine and guide you. However, when the diet is in harmony with the ketone (i.e., allergen & toxin free), you do not need to do any calorie restriction.

Number 4-

I used *Self* magazine's website (http://nutritiondata.self.com) to provide nutrition facts for food items that don't come with labels (to be able to calculate total fat, proteins and total carbohydrates per serving size). You can search this site for any food.

There are also various publications that can be used for carbohydrate gram counting and there are various free applications that can be easily downloaded on cell phones.

Number 5-

If you start the diet with a fast (as in not eating for twenty-four hours), then you will get ketone after approximately twenty-four hours. If you start the diet without fasting and eat food, you will get ketone after approximately forty-eight hours. This is how long it will take you to deplete the sugar reserves that are stored in your body. After you've depleted the glucose you will start having ketone in your urine. Therefore, it is not worth checking ketone until after twenty-four hours if you fasted or forty-eight hours if you are eating, because it will probably be negative and you will just waste testing strips.

Number 6-

Both Dr. John M. Freeman's book and the Spanish Mediterranean ketogenic diet advise to take supplements while on a ketogenic diet such as a multivitamin (I take organic only); extra calcium and vitamin D (Dr. Mercola recommends D3 along with K2); potassium citrate; carnitine; omega-3 fatty acids (you can get some in fish if you eat fish or from parent essential oils); selenium; and magnesium. In case of constipation, use MCT oil, eat avocados, and drink more water. Some of the supplements prevent kidney stones by raising the urine pH to be more alkaline (such as potassium citrate). Leg cramps might indicate low magnesium so these are important. If you take the supplements and still have leg cramps, eating might help. It should go away within 30 minutes after eating. As well, drinking plenty of the permitted fluids is good for the kidneys.

Number 7-

My lump started decreasing from approximately day 7 to 14 on the diet, so if I had stayed on the diet for only a week, it would not have been enough (it also takes up to forty-eight hours to deplete the glucose that fuels the cancer, so it takes about up to three days to take away the cancer's fuel). Also, at about the same time my lump started decreasing, I started having aches, pains and suction-like feelings. It is normal. Other people doing my diet also report the same thing with tumor pain when cancer starts to shrink.

Number 8-

For diabetics, the blood glucose *must* be kept under 200 mg/dl, to be on the safe side, at all time on this diet. Levels below 70mg/dl would be optimal for cancer. Ketones protect against hypoglycemia adverse effects.

Number 9-

I did not do any calorie restriction while on this diet and I did not do any liquid intake restriction either. I had as much food as I needed and I drank as much as I needed. I just made sure every time I put something in my mouth to drink or eat that it either had zero total carbs or had at least a minimum 3:1 ratio (i.e., [Protein+Fat]: [Total Carbs]) to 5:1 ratio. My weight stayed stable, my skin became soft, and my energy level went up.

Number 10-

I used a water filter and I also used a device to make my water alkaline. I added things to it to increase its alkalinity, such as lemon, mint or wheatgrass powder. I also drank mineral water. For forty-nine dollars, my filter removes chlorine, lead, mercury, pharmaceuticals, microbial cysts, industrial chemicals (asbestos and benzene), agricultural pollutants (pesticides and herbicides), and chlorination by-products (TTHM).

Number 11-

How do you read food labels? You need to look at portion size/serving size; total fat; total carbohydrates; protein; calories (if you want to for weight maintenance, gain, or loss), and all ingredients.

Here are some examples to help understand food labels (for demonstration purposes only, as I would not eat some of these things on my ketogenic diet version).

In this first food label example, for 1 cup of this food, you have total of fat plus protein of 1gram (i.e., 0+1=1) and you have total carbohydrates of 10gr. To be ketogenic, you need at least a 3:1 ratio of fat+protein compared to carbs, and in this example, you have a 1:10 ratio, which is not ketogenic at all.

Now if you only eat one-fourth of the cup, by dividing by four you now have less than 1gram of fat+protein and 2.5 grams of total carbohydrates. So now you have a <1: 2.5 ratio and to make it ketogenic, you need to add something that contains only fat or protein that is at least three to five times the amount of carbs. Therefore 2.5 x 3 = 7.5 grams, which means you need to add something that contains at least 7.5 grams of fat and protein combined (or just from fat, or just from protein), to make it ketogenic

Nutrition Facts

Serving Size 1 cup (85g) (3 oz.)

Servings per container 2.5

Amount per serving

Calories 45   Calories from Fat 0

	% Daily Value*
Total Fat 0g	0%
Saturated Fat 0g	0%
Cholesterol 0mg	0%
Sodium 55 mg	2%
Total Carbohydrate 10g	3%
Dietary Fiber 3g	12%
Sugars 5g	
Protein 1g	

Vitamin A 350% • Vitamin C 8% • Calcium 2% • Iron 0%

*Percent Daily Values are based on a 2,000 calorie diet. Your daily values may be higher or lower depending on your calorie needs.

	Calories	2,000	2,500
Total Fat	Less than	65g	80g
Sat Fat	Less than	20g	25g
Cholesterol	Less than	300mg	300mg
Sodium	Less than	2,400mg	2,400mg
Total Carbohydrate	Less than	300mg	375mg
Dietary Fiber	Less than	25g	30g

Calories per gram Fat 9 • Carbohydrate 4 • Protein 4

Ingredients: Carrots

In the second example, for 2 crackers, you have fat + protein that equal 2+1.5=3.5 grams for 10grams of total carbs. Again, this is not ketogenic, because you have a 3.5:10 ratio.

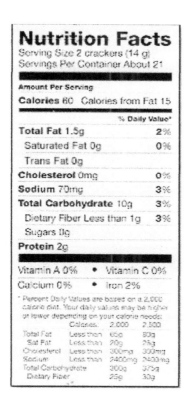

In the ingredients list, "Flavoring" or "natural flavoring" can be anything, so avoid that as it can hide an allergen.

The third example is for food ingredients. I am off dairy, and this has dairy. I do not eat any vegetable oil that says "hydrogenated" (a chemical process that extends shelf life), and this has some, on top of being a bad, unhealthy source of fat. It has soy and I do not eat any soy. It is not ketogenic either, because 12 + 10=22 for 24 grams of carbs makes a 22:24 ratio. It also says that it has flavoring but does not say from what source.

Nutrition Facts	Amount/serving	%DV*	Amount/serving	%DV*
Serv. Size 1 cup (249g)	Total Fat 12g	18%	Sodium 940mg	39%
	Sat. Fat 6g	30%	Total Carb. 24g	8%
Servings About 2	Polyunsat. Fat 1.5g		Dietary Fiber 1g	4%
Calories 250 Fat Cal. 110	Monounsat. Fat 2.5g		Sugars 1g	
*Percent Daily Values (DV) are based on a 2,000 calorie diet.	Cholest. 60mg	20%	Protein 10g	20%
	Vitamin A 0% • Vitamin C 0% • Calcium 6% • Iron 8%			

Ingredients: Water, chicken stock, enriched pasta semolina, wheat, flour, egg white solids, niacin, iron, thiamine, mononitrate (vitamin B1), riboflavin (vitamin B2) and folic acid, Cream (derived from milk), chicken, contains less than 2% of cheeses (granular, parmesan and romano paste, pasteurized cow's milk, cultures, salt enzymes, water, salt, lactic acid, citric acid and disodium phosphate. Butter pasteurized sweet cream (derived from milk). Modified corn starch, salt, whole egg solids, sugar, rice starch, datem, garlic, spice, xanthan gum, cheese flavor, partially hydrogenated soybean oil, flavorings and smoke flavoring. Mustard flour, isolated soy protein and sodium phosphate.

Serving Size: 1 oz • 28g • 30 pieces	
Amount Per Serving	
Calories 170	Calories from Fat 130
	% DV
Total Fat 15g	23%
Saturated Fat 2g	10%
Trans Fat 0g	
Polyunsaturated Fat 4g	
Monounsaturated Fat 8g	
Cholesterol 0mg	0%
Sodium 110mg	5%
Potassium 190mg	5%
Total Carbohydrate 5g	2%
Dietary Fiber 2g	8%
Sugars 1g	
Protein 6g	12%

Vitamin A 0%	•	Vitamin C 0%
Calcium 2%	•	Iron 8%
Vitamin E 15%	•	Niacin 10%
Phosphorus 15%	•	Magnesium 15%
Copper 20%	•	Manganese 30%

Now this last example is for a particular brand of mixed nuts that is ketogenic due its ratio. For 1 ounce, it has 15 grams of fat + 6 grams of protein= (21 grams) and it has 5 grams of total carbs. Thus, a 21:5 ratio. If we simplify it, this means approximately 4:1 ratio. That is something that I would eat.

CHAPTER ELEVEN:

Recipes

We have drifted so far from eating a healthy diet – for some people, even their grandparents may also have grown up eating microwaved foods, pizza, chips, and donuts, so the experience of real food has been almost completely lost.

Changing from the standard American diet (SAD) is challenging because people don't know how to prepare food or what foods are particularly healthy. The amount of sugar in our diets has gone from 20 teaspoons in a year to 50 teaspoons in a day!

The good news is that millions of people have succeeded in dieting using very similar principles to these. So they found it possible to stick to a very low carb diet, and so can you. There are many tricks that will help you make the transition to a much healthier way of eating, so you can help your body to heal itself.

Because the diet is so high in healthy fat and proteins and so full of good nutrition, you won't go hungry.

GUIDELINES

- If it's not recognizable to you as something that once ran, swam, or grew, it's likely your body won't recognize it either. Buy your foods from the fruit and vegetable section and the refrigerated section of your supermarket. The parts of the supermarket that contain the healthiest food seem to be the departments located around the perimeter of the store. All the shelves in the middle contain manufactured and processed goods (unless they have designated organic sections), so the easiest way to avoid temptation is just to walk around the perimeter of the store and look for the organic section.

- Throw out all your processed vegetable oils, butter, and margarines- that means corn oil, canola, soy oil, sunflower seed oil, and any products containing them. The latest research indicates that because these oils are heat-treated so many times during manufacturing they actually are very difficult for the body to use properly, so they lead to illness rather than health. The Indian Medical Association published a paper in 1998 advising that their research suggested that the rising rate of heart disease and type 2 diabetes in the Indian population over the last fifty years was due to using processed vegetable oils instead of their traditional cooking oils, such as ghee, coconut oil, and mustard seed oil. They recommended a return to the traditional oils that our ancestors safely used for thousands of years. As well, per Andrew Kimbrell in the movie *The Beautiful Truth*, there are four GMO crops in the USA and they are corn, canola, soy, and cotton. He said that GMO crop food can be toxic and the FDA has admitted that GMO crops can create new allergens. Canola oil is therefore prohibited on my diet. The oils permitted in my diet are non-GMO and are not the commonly used vegetable oils, which are high in omega-6 ratios that show links to inflammation, cancer, and type II diabetes.

- Use extra-virgin olive Oil for baking and salad dressings. Extra-virgin olive oil is healthy because it is not processed. It is squeezed out of olives, strained, and bottled. It's as close to natural as you can get without making your own.

- Use coconut oil and eat 4 to 6 tablespoons throughout the day to adjust ketone rapidly, and for cooking, etc. Recent research has shown that coconut oil is actually an extremely healthy fat containing many beneficial ingredients. For years patients in intensive care units and premature babies have been fed medical-grade foods containing coconut oil because of its easy digestibility and superior nutrition. Consider that South Sea Islanders were considered the most perfect examples of human beauty and perfection and their diet contains 50 to 60 percent of coconut. If that diet was unhealthy, surely they would have died out generations ago? Coconut oil is high in the kinds of fats that make up your brain, and research in the last few years suggests it can be helpful in all times of memory deterioration, including pregnancy, the "fluffy brain" that many women have experienced, middle-aged absent-mindedness, and has even shown benefit for restoring function for patients with Alzheimer's, Parkinson's, MS and other disorders. Coconut oil is naturally high in medium-chain triglycerides (MCT) which are broken down in the body into ketones. Dr. Mary Newport and Dr. Veech have extensive research on this and on ketone ester.[113] [114]

- Get rid of all the sugar and products containing sugar, fructose (including fresh fruits), and ideally all artificial sweeteners as well. One product that didn't even exist before 1980 is called high fructose corn syrup and now it's included in thousands of manufactured goods, both sweet and savoury. People think because it is fruit sugar that it has to be better for you, but sadly, no.

TRICKS

- At least in the beginning use sugar replacements if you are craving sugar. Stevia is recommended, as it is a completely natural product. Make sure you use the pure stevia extract, not the little sachets of powder that usually contain some kind of powdered sugar and will add to your daily carbohydrate total.

- Use ready-bagged salads, jars of black olives, and tins of anchovies, herrings, and sardines. You can use mayonnaise, raw coconut oil, nuts, and cacao butter if you need to add fat and to up the calorie intake.

- You can also make homemade almond milk in a high-speed blender using three cups of water for one cup of almonds. You can also buy unsweetened coconut milk or almond milk.

The following section is for recipes. They are provided to give you ideas of things you can eat on my diet. They are recipes I make for my family and to have leftovers to bring for lunch at work.

Therefore, you will need to count carbs and figure out the portion sizes.

As I mentioned previously, there are various carb counting resources available (i.e., books, websites, and cell phone applications that can be downloaded for free).

For those who don't want to count carbs, you can eat only foods that are only sources of fat and proteins using herbs, spices, lemon, garlic, and onions for seasoning.

Here are some examples of foods that are only sources of fat and proteins, and that you can eat as much as you want of: chicken, turkey, eggs, fish, seafood, raw cacao butter, olive oil, coconut oil, and mayonnaise.

EXAMPLES OF HEALTHY LOW CARB RECIPES I USED

VINAIGRETTES:

Quick Simple Balsamic Vinaigrette:

3 parts olive oil

1 part balsamic vinegar

Garlic to taste

Healthy salt (with iodine) and pepper

In liquid measure or small bowl, whisk together all ingredients; shake well. Refrigerate in an airtight container for up to three days.

Balsamic Vinaigrette

3/4 cup extra-virgin olive oil

1/3 cup balsamic vinegar

1 tablespoon lemon juice

1 teaspoon Dijon mustard

1 clove garlic, minced

1/4 teaspoon healthy salt

1/4 teaspoon pepper

In liquid measure or small bowl, whisk together all ingredients. Refrigerate in an airtight container for up to three days.

Use your imagination combo

I buy a sun dried tomato and garlic organic vinaigrette that is also gluten free (with o gram of sugar & total carbs <1g per two tablespoon; it has no fat and no proteins). I mix it with some extra-virgin olive oil to add fat to it. You can add basil or garlic to taste.

You can use your imagination to make any combination that pleases you, as long as it's healthy and has ingredients that don't hurt your body.

Salad dressing

Tahini and basil makes a great combination for a dressing. Tahini is a paste made from sesame seeds and is a good source of calcium. It's high in good fats and protein. Thin it down with some extra-virgin olive oil. Add a bit of healthy sea salt and maybe some garlic to taste. It's a very rich creamy dressing.

LOW CARB MAYONNAISE

Mayonnaise can be used in salads, as a dip, or as topping for fish.

A) Olive oil mayonnaise (optional with Dijon mustard). Look for the one that has the fewer carbs, or you can make it homemade with olive oil and eggs, plus add any other healthy ingredients to taste. YouTube is a great reference for videos that show you how to make homemade mayonnaise.

B) Olive oil mayonnaise with lemon juice and garlic with healthy salt and pepper. You can replace the lemon by capers for fish and you can add black olives for turkey.

FAT & PROTEIN SNACKS:

Black olives

Mixed nuts, peanuts, and almonds

Organic low-carb raw seaweeds from Maine (approximately 3 grams of total carbs per 1/3 of a cup).

Hard-boiled eggs

Sardines, trout or herring with fresh lemon juice

Protein shake (17grams proteins, 1.2 gram fat and
1 gram total carbs)

OVEN BAKED FISH:

This recipe can be used with any fish, such as salmon, haddock, sole, cod, tilapia, trout, etc. (you can also fry in pan with olive oil to add fat)

Fresh Salmon fish filets

Extra-virgin olive oil

Basil

Parsley

Healthy salt and pepper

Turmeric/curcumin

Cajun spices/ or Jamaica allspice (optional) or seafood spices (optional)

Garlic

Lemon juice

Onions slices or mushrooms

Place the fish in a baking pan with a little olive oil at the bottom. Add the ingredients to taste. Bake at 350 degrees for 30 to 40 minutes, until fish flakes easily with fork.

TURKEY PATTIES OR MEATBALLS

(patties or meat balls)

Fresh ground turkey

Extra-virgin olive oil

1 onion, diced

Basil

Parsley

Cayenne pepper (tiny amount) or Jamaican
    allspice

Healthy salt & pepper

Turmeric/curcumin

Cajun spices (optional)

Garlic

In a skillet over medium heat, sauté onion first in olive oil. In a bowl, combine remaining ingredients. Form into patties or meat-balls. Cook in skillet, adding more olive oil or coconut oil if desired, until meatballs are cooked through.

CILANTRO CHICKEN

Cilantro (also called coriander leaf) is known to help with the detoxification of metals like mercury and lead.

Fresh chicken breasts (whole or cut in pieces)

Fresh lemon juice (3 to 4 lemons)

Healthy salt & pepper

Turmeric/curcumin

One onion sliced

Fresh cilantro to taste

In a skillet, sauté all ingredients in a pan with coconut oil or olive oil until the chicken is cooked through.

TURMERIC CHICKEN

6 fresh chicken breasts, cubed

Handful of Basil, chopped

Handful of Parsley, chopped

Cayenne pepper to taste

Sea salt and pepper

Turmeric/curcumin

1 onion sliced

Organic or homemade chicken broth

1 cup water

Red peppers (optional)

Garlic

Coconut oil or olive oil

In a skillet, sauté all ingredients in oil until the chicken is cooked through.

Chicken Drumsticks With Lemon Slices and Herbs.

Recipe taken from: Every Day Health.
<http://www.everydayhealth.com/weight/chicken-drumsticks-with-lemon-and-herbs.aspx>
Originally from: Suzanne Somers Sexy Forever.

8 medium chicken drumsticks

8 teaspoons extra-virgin olive oil

1/2 teaspoon sea salt

1/2 teaspoon freshly ground black pepper

7 cloves of garlic

2-1/2 cups of mixed fresh herbs (thyme, rosemary, tarragon, sage, or parsley)

2 medium lemons cut into thin slices

Preheat oven to 350 degrees.

Place the drumsticks in a large roasting pan. Generously drizzle with olive oil, then season with sea salt, pepper, garlic, and fresh herbs.

Place lemon slices on top of each drumstick and the leftovers on the bottom of the pan.

Place the pan in the oven and cook for about 80 minutes.

While roasting, turn drumsticks and scrape the lemon slices from the bottom of the pan from time to time to loosen and evenly brown.

Serve the drumsticks with the cooked lemon slices and crispy herbs.

BOILED CHICKEN:

3 big chicken breasts
1 teaspoon of thyme
3 onions diced
1 tablespoon garlic
A little pinch of Cayenne pepper
Healthy sea salt and pepper
Fresh cilantro
Any other Italian seasoning (to taste)

Put everything in a pot and add water to cover the chicken (you can also use organic chicken or veggie broth or a mix). Put a lid on and bring to a boil (5-10 minutes). When it comes to a boil, turn down the heat to 4 and open the lid a little so the steam can come out. Cook slowly for 2 to 2.5 hours.

The broth can be eaten as a soup. The chicken can be mixed with mayonnaise to make chicken salad.

SPINACH OMELETTE or SCRAMBLED EGGS

4 to 6 eggs

A bit of water to fluff (1/3 cup maximum)

Healthy salt and pepper

Spinach, shredded

Mushrooms, sliced

Parsley

Basil

Garlic (optional)

Paprika

Extra-virgin olive oil

In a bowl, beat eggs; add remaining ingredients except oil. Add a little bit of olive oil to a sauté pan over high heat. Pour egg mixture into pan.

For omelette: as eggs set, take a spatula and lift the edges of the egg mixture, allowing the uncooked eggs on top to flow underneath. Repeat the procedure at various spots around the edge. Then reduce the heat to low; continue to cook until the eggs are cooked through.

For scrambled eggs: reduce heat to low and stir constantly. Remove to plate when eggs are set.

GARLIC SHRIMPS

1 to 2 lbs. shrimp, cleaned
Coconut oil or olive oil
Garlic
Parsley
Fresh lemon juice (optional)

In a pan, sauté shrimp in oil; add garlic and parsley to taste. Cook until shrimp turn pink. You can also drizzle with fresh lemon juice if desired.

Note: do not use the lemon concentrate containing sulfites.

ANTI-INFLAMMATORY LEMONADE

1 cup fresh squeezed lemon juice (4 to 6 lemons)

4 to 6 cups of filtered water

1 teaspoon ground turmeric

1 teaspoon cinnamon

Pinch of healthy salt with iodine

1/2 teaspoon of natural stevia to sweeten (if desired)

Optional: 1 teaspoon ground or fresh ginger, chopped

Mix together with some ice and serve with mint leaves or a slice of lemon.

BROCCOLI SALAD WITH AVOCADO

Cut a slice off the butt end of each large broccoli stalk and peel the stalks just below the outer fibrous layer.

1 pound broccoli

1 ripe avocado

2 tablespoons extra virgin olive oil

2 tablespoons freshly squeezed lemon juice

1 tablespoon grainy prepared mustard

Trim and wash the broccoli. Cut it into bite-sized pieces. Steam or boil until it is just crisp-tender; drain and cool.

Peel and pit the avocado. Cut it into small cubes. Fold avocado into the broccoli.

Whisk together olive oil, lemon juice, and mustard. Toss the broccoli and avocado with the dressing.

ELAINE CANTIN

EASY ROASTED ASPARAGUS

My favourite way to eat this yummy vegetable, which contains vitamin D, folic acid, and the antioxidant glutathione.

Asparagus

Extra-virgin olive oil

Healthy sea salt

Fresh minced garlic or garlic powder

Fresh lemon juice

Trim fresh asparagus about an inch from the bottom hard part. Place in a baking pan.
Drizzle with olive oil; toss. Add sea salt and fresh garlic or garlic powder to taste; toss.
Bake at 350 degrees for about 30 minutes, or until crisp-tender. Before serving, drizzle with fresh lemon juice.

KALE

Bag of fresh kale

1 onion, sliced

Healthy sea salt and black pepper

Extra-virgin olive oil

Fresh garlic or garlic powder to taste

Rosemary

Turmeric/curcumin

Fresh lemon juice and lemon zest

In a sauté pan, cook kale and onion in olive oil; season to taste.

SPINACH SAUTÉ

1 lb. container fresh organic spinach

Extra-virgin olive oil

Healthy salt and pepper

Fresh lemon juice

Garlic

In a sauté pan, cook spinach in olive oil; season to taste.

MARINATED TURKEY STRIPS

Turkey breast, cut into small strips
Extra-virgin olive oil
Cumin
Turmeric
Cardamom
Coriander/cilantro
Paprika
Black pepper and sea salt
Chili powder
Ginger
Curry leaves
Cinnamon

Combine turkey strips, olive oil, and spices. Cover and marinate for one hour to overnight. Bake at 350 degrees for about 30 to 45 minutes.

Serving suggestion: Dip in a black olive mayonnaise dip (see mayonnaise dip recipes).

MARINATED CHICKEN

Chicken breasts

Extra-virgin olive oil

Garlic

Turmeric

Coriander/cilantro

Black pepper and healthy sea salt

Lemon, sliced

Fresh spinach

Combine all ingredients except chicken and spinach in a bowl. Add chicken; cover and marinate for two hours to overnight. Bake slowly so it is soft, tender and moist. Serve over Spinach.

OVEN ROASTED AUBERGINE (Eggplant)

One baby aubergine, sliced into thirds.

Garlic powder

Extra-virgin olive oil

Healthy salt

Parsley

Sprinkle slices with garlic powder, a little olive oil, salt, and parsley. Bake at 350 degrees for approximately 25 minutes, until tender.

Almond Flour muffins

2 cups almond flour/almond meal

2 teaspoons baking powder

1/4 teaspoon healthy salt

1/2 cup extra-virgin olive oil or coconut oil

4 eggs

1/3 cup water or alkaline water

Stevia to taste -- about 1/3 cup (liquid might be better; use natural stevia)

Walnuts or mixed spices to taste

Mix all ingredients. Fill cups of an oiled muffin tin 2/3 full. Bake at 350 degrees for about 15 minutes, or until muffins test done with a toothpick.

ALMOND MILK

For healthier almond milk, soak almonds overnight, drain and blend with fresh water.

For super-healthy almond milk follow the directions above but let stand in a warm place for two days before putting in the refrigerator. This allows fermenting to begin which breaks down the almonds, making them even more digestible.

Super Quick Almond Milk

Mix 1 cup of almonds and 3 cups of filtered water in a high-speed blender; blend on high speed until fully combined. Note: by soaking the almonds, you remove most of the lectins.

ALMOND BUTTER

Place 1 cup of almonds in a blender; blend on high speed until almonds form a buttery/grainy paste (if desired you can add a little olive oil).

Cumin Shrimps

Extra-virgin olive oil

Juice of 2 lemons

1 to 2 onions, sliced

1 tablespoon cumin

2-3 lbs frozen shrimps

Garlic optional (to taste)

Combine all ingredients in a large sauce pan; cover and and cook over high heat for three to five minutes, or until shrimps are pink and cooked through.

Chicken Kebabs

½ lbs. Chicken, cubed

2 tablespoons red wine vinegar

½ teaspoon healthy salt

½ teaspoon red pepper flakes

1 tablespoon extra- virgin olive oil

1 tablespoon basil

1 tablespoon oregano

2 garlic cloves

Zucchini, cubed

Whole mushrooms

Red or yellow peppers, cubed

Combine all ingredients in a plastic zip-top bag; marinate for no longer than 15 minutes. Thread chicken and veggies on wooden skewers. Bake at 400 degrees for 15 to 20 minutes, or until chicken fully cooked.

Avocado Soup

1 cup of filtered water

1 avocado, cut into chunks

1 to 2 cloves of garlic

1 teaspoon of red pepper flakes

1 tablespoon fresh lemon juice

Healthy salt and pepper

Put all ingredients (except garnish) in a blender; process on high speed for one to two minutes. Garnish with red onions and alfalfa sprouts, if desired.

Marinated Tilapia (or other fish)

Tilapia filets

Garlic

1 teaspoon cumin

Cayenne pepper

1 cup fresh lemon juice

Combine all ingredients except fish; add fish and marinate in the fridge for one hour. Cook filets in a sauté pan over low heat in olive oil, until fish flakes with a fork. Discard remaining marinade.

Low-Carb Pancakes Recipe:

1 cup almond meal or almond flour

2 eggs

1/4 cup water (for puffier pancakes, you can use sparkling water)

2 to 3 tablespoons coconut oil

1/4 teaspoon salt

1 teaspoon stevia

Garnish: fresh lemon juice, stevia, sugar-free maple syrup with zero carbs.

Mix ingredients together and cook as you would other pancakes. I like to use a non-stick pan with a little oil. The only real difference is that they won't "bubble" on top the same way as regular pancakes. Flip them when the underside is brown. For garnish you can use fresh lemon juice with stevia or sugar-free maple syrup with zero carbs.

Make sure you use almond flour that has at least three times the fat plus proteins compared to carbs: 100 grams of almonds have 84 grams of fat+protein and 16 grams Carbohydrates. Therefore, fresh-ground almonds are naturally ketogenic. Check the ingredients of any pre-packaged almond meal or almond flour to ensure they have the same ratios.

Ketogenic Protein Shakes

These can be made with unsweetened almond milk or unsweetened coconut milk. Filtered water can also be used instead of the non-dairy-milk.

Look for raw protein powder, that is plant based with a complete amino acid profile that is gluten-free, soy-free, Dairy-free, non-GMO, hypo-allergenic, and fortified with coconut (MCT) oil. Made with: pea protein, cranberry protein, hemp protein, and medium chain triglycerides (MCT).

The protein powder that I use has only 1 gram of total carbohydrates, 1.2 grams of total fat, and 17 grams of protein per scoop.

Mix well with non-dairy milk or water; refrigerate and serve.

Note: you can also add stevia or cinnamon to the taste.

Some spices have carbohydrates – e.g., 1 teaspoon cinnamon = 2 grams carbs, so it needs to be factored into your 20 to 30 grams of total carbs per day.

Kale Chips

You can also make them in a food dehydrator if you prefer.

A bunch of fresh kale, stems removed
Extra-virgin olive oil
Turmeric
Pepper and healthy sea salt
Garlic to taste (optional)

Chop or tear kale into large pieces. Drizzle olive oil on a baking sheet; place kale on top. Sprinkle with: turmeric, pepper, healthy sea salt, olive oil. Add garlic (optional).

Bake at 350 degrees for 10 to 15 minutes, until crisp.

Low-Carb Muffins

2 cups almond flour

3 eggs

¼ teaspoon salt

¼ cup water

¼ cup olive oil or coconut oil

Sweetener to taste (use natural stevia)

For additional flavour, use a handful of walnuts or 1 teaspoon mixed spices

Mix all ingredients; fill 8 muffin greased muffin cups 2/3 full. Bake at 350 degrees for 20 minutes, or until muffins test done with a toothpick.

Almond Crackers

1 cup almond flour

1 egg white

Sea salt

Mix all ingredients; add filtered water and spices to taste-garlic/onion powder, crushed red pepper, cayenne pepper, etc. Line cookie sheet with parchment paper and roll out mixture as thin as you like by placing a piece of wax paper on top. Score the crackers by using a pizza cutter. Put sea salt on top. Bake at 325 degrees for approximately 10 minutes. The edges will brown first so you can remove them and place the rest back in the oven. Watch closely and remove the edges as they brown. After they are cooled they are ready to eat or to be stored.

Non Dairy Sour Cream

1 cup of soaked raw cashews

1 cup of water

1 teaspoon of vitamin C powder

¼ teaspoon sea salt

Soak cashews for 2 hours in water. Blend all ingredients in a food processor till smooth. Add more water for desired consistency. Chill for about 30 minutes- it will thicken a little when chilled.

You can also serve mixing with 1 tablespoon of dried basil, 2 teaspoons of fresh lemon juice, dill, lemon thyme, etc...

Low Carb Bread

16 once creamy almond butter

6 eggs

¾ cup warm filtered water

2 teaspoons baking powder

1 packet stevia (optional)

1/2 teaspoon sea salt

Mix eggs and almond butter until smooth. Add all other ingredients. Pour into a greased 9" X 5" loaf pan and smooth on top. Bake at 325 degrees for about 60 minutes. Let it cool before slicing. You can also use muffin tins for buns.

***How to make almond butter:

Place 1 cup of almonds in a blender; blend on high speed until almonds form a buttery/grainy paste (if desired you can add a little olive oil).

Boiled Lobster or Crab Legs

Submerge the lobster(s) or crab legs in boiling water that has some healthy salt in it.

Lobster: Boil up to 2 pounds lobster for approximately up to 10 minutes, 2 to 4 pounds up to 15 minutes, or until the entire shell is red.

King Crab from Alaska: soak and rinse before boiling. Boil for 7 to 10 minutes.

Snow crab: soak and rinse before boiling. Boil for approximately 7 minutes.

Dip in a fresh lemon juice mixed with minced garlic or mayonnaise.

Jerk Chicken (or pork)

Ingredients:

Jerk seasoning
Olive oil
Chicken spices
Chicken cut in small cubes
Fresh lime juice
Sea salt and pepper

Marinate in the refrigerator overnight all the ingredients. In a sauté pan, cook in olive oil until chicken fully cooked. Serve with slices of fresh lime.

Marinated Cod or Haddock

Ingredients:

Cod or haddock fillets
Fresh Parsley
Olive oil
Garlic
Fresh lime juice
Fish spices

Marinate in the refrigerator overnight all the ingredients. In a sauté pan, cook in olive oil until fish flakes with a fork. Serve with slices of fresh lime.

DAILY MENUS EXAMPLES

	DAY 1
Breakfast	Fried egg(s); natural turkey sausage; sliced fresh avocado.
Morning Snack	Mixed nuts
Lunch	Cilantro chicken; fresh spinach
Afternoon Snack	Seaweeds
Dinner	Oven-baked salmon; roasted asparagus.

	DAY 2
Breakfast	Spinach and mushroom omelette
Morning Snack	Black olives
Lunch	Fried tilapia; steamed cauliflower
Afternoon Snack	Cinnamon-coated almonds
Dinner	Marinated chicken on bed of fresh spinach

	DAY 3
Breakfast	Scrambled eggs, sliced fresh avocado
Morning Snack	Almonds
Lunch	Cumin shrimps; roasted asparagus
Afternoon Snack	Black olives
Dinner	Turmeric chicken; steamed broccoli

	DAY 4
Breakfast	Poached eggs; fried onions; natural sausage
Morning Snack	Cinnamon-coated almonds
Lunch	Turkey meat balls; fresh spinach
Afternoon Snack	Mixed nuts
Dinner	Oven-baked haddock; sautéed kale

	DAY 5
Breakfast	Spinach and mushroom omelette
Morning Snack	Black olives
Lunch	Garlic shrimps; mixed salad
Afternoon Snack	Cinnamon-coated almonds
Dinner	Cilantro chicken; Brussels sprouts

	DAY 6
Breakfast	Fried egg(s); natural turkey sausage; sliced onions
Morning Snack	Mixed nuts
Lunch	Jerk chicken; broccoli
Afternoon Snack	Seaweeds
Dinner	Turkey patties; watercress salad

	DAY 7
Breakfast	Scrambled eggs, sliced fresh avocado
Morning Snack	Sardines with fresh lemon juice
Lunch	Fried salmon; mushrooms
Afternoon Snack	Cinnamon- coated almonds
Dinner	Chicken Drum sticks; sautéed spinach

CHAPTER TWELVE

Emergency Brain Surgery

On March 9, 2012, my sister had to go through emergency brain surgery due to a brain aneurism.

After a long surgery, the surgeon informed us that she was critical for the next seventy-two hours. We were told she might not survive. They planned to keep her in a coma for as long as needed, to keep the pressure in her brain stable in order to avoid additional bleeding.

If she survived, she would have to have another surgery later to put back a section of skull bone from the back of the left side of her head, which was taken out during surgery and left out because of swelling.

We were told her eye-sight would be affected because of where the bleeding was, and she would possibly have other issues that would remain unknown until she woke up, if she survived. The bleeding was like an inch and a half, so there would probably be other issues.

She survived the surgery and she survived the seventy-two-hours period after surgery. For the next 5 to 6 days after the surgery, she was kept in a coma. We just kept praying.

When she woke up from the coma, it was like she had dementia. She would stare at the ceiling and start talking about random things. She did not make any sense. She was unable to move her right arm and right leg. Her right foot was like pointed inward and her right hand was curled up toward her body. She is right-handed and she could not even hold a fork.

When I saw her with this blank stare, it reminded me of my grandma who had Alzheimer's. Right away this made me think about my own research and the information I had found that connected coconut oil and ketones to help patients with Alzheimer's disease. It reminded me that I had read somewhere that ketones were the best source of fuel for the brain, and about the video I had seen from Dr. Mary Newport and her husband who had experienced improvement with Alzheimer's.[115]

The hospital staff was trying to make her eat and drink to get her off the IV fluid and the urine bag. I looked at the food closely and it was some kind of sweet pudding. There was also some sort of vanilla drink. I looked at the ingredients on the drink label and it was loaded with sugar and all sorts of artificial ingredients.
When they would try to put the food in her mouth, she would spit it back out. I remember

thinking to myself that this was not something healthy and it was good she was rejecting it.

I left the hospital and went directly to get organic pure coconut oil and unsweetened almond milk. I remembered reading that almonds have zinc, which is good for the brain, on top of other nutrients; they are also low in carbohydrates. I begged my family to feed her these two things and to shove the coconut oil down her throat if they had to. I reminded them that everyone thought I was crazy when I refused all conventional cancer treatments and did my diet instead. I told them to look at me now and I reminded them I was in complete remission because of my diet. I told them that I loved my sister and I wanted her to get better and they needed to trust me because I was certain this would help her. I insisted so much that they did it. Right after waking up from coma, after they removed the tube from her mouth, she was fed the coconut oil and the unsweetened almond milk.

When she started eating more, my mom would send homemade food to the hospital for her and she was fed coconut oil three times per day.

Within a couple of days, she was talking and started to make more sense. Next her right foot and the right arm started working. Soon, she could walk. The staff in intermediate care could not believe the progress she was making so quickly. My sister did not like the taste of the coconut oil, but I told her that I did not care if she did not like it, and that I wanted her to promise me she would take it because I loved her and I wanted her to get better. She promised and she was taking it three times per day with her food. Since she did not have the skull section replaced yet, she had someone watching her 24/7 so that she would not bump her head and die. The hospital staffs (even doctors) were asking her what she was eating when she was eating her huge spoonfuls of greasy coconut oil and grimacing. She would tell them it was for her brain and she had promised her sister she would take it. They would look at her jar and say "yuk" or not say a word and let her have it.

She stayed a month in intermediate care due to not having the skull section to protect the brain. After a month, she had another surgery to replace the bone. The anaesthetist that came to see her before surgery was the same one from the first surgery. He was looking at her file, he told her she was coming from far and that he could not believe how well she was doing after what she had gone through.

A couple of days after the second surgery, she was released to a rehab place. At the rehab place, they did not know what to do with her. She was the only one walking and not paralyzed; she could wash herself, she could feed herself; she could put her clothes on; and she was walking in her high-heeled sandals-she wanted nothing to do with the "ugly shoes" they recommended and she did not even need them. She was told that people who had half the bleeding on their brains that she had were paralyzed and they could not believe how well she was doing. After only a couple of days, she was released and sent home.

At home, they sent someone to follow up with her. My sister told the rehab worker who came to her house that she was not able to go on the Internet and type on the keyboard. She was told to forget about that, as she would no longer be able to write and type and she just needed to adjust to her new reality. Two days later, my sister started typing and sent me a message online. I started crying when I received her message...very happy tears.

In the book *"The Ketogenic Diets,"*[116] there is a list of non epileptic conditions that new evidence shows the ketogenic diet may be beneficial for. The list includes the following conditions: brain tumours and perhaps other cancers; severe head trauma and perhaps hypoxic/ischemic encephalopathy; stroke; heart disease; Alzheimer's disease; Parkinson's disease; amyotrophic lateral sclerosis (ALS); diabetes; autism; inflammatory disease; migraine; severe hyperactivity; and other diseases.

My sister keeps taking her coconut oil and maintains a low-carb diet. She keeps doing better and better. Coincidence? I don't think so!

EPILOGUE

This research was done with my heart fully in it. The knowledge I acquired for my son also probably saved my life when I was diagnosed with an aggressive form of cancer.

I am passing this knowledge along, hoping it will help you with your health. I hope you will learn, just like I did, how powerful the food we eat is.

If needed, you can find a support group for my diet at the following link: http://www.facebook.com/#!/groups/ElaineAltern ativeHealthTips/?bookmark_t=group. It is called Elaine's alternative tips for cancer, type I diabetes & other ailments.

Again, because it is worth the emphasis, I hope you will never underestimate the power of food from now on. From my heart, I wish upon you health, love and blessings. Just like the title of Mr. Abrahams' movie says, and especially for the little kids and the ones who are suffering, I leave you with these appropriate words: "FIRST DO NO HARM".

TESTIMONIALS

I was doing pretty badly. My tumors were crushing my trachea, throat, left lung and aorta. It had gotten to the point where I had to sleep sitting up and I would wake up at night because I couldn't breathe. My pills were also getting stuck in my throat and hurt really bad. I had chemo, and radiation and I tried alternative therapies but nothing worked.

I started switching over to Elaine Cantin's diet. I finally got the diet down without messing it up. Within the first week and a half, from what I can measure around my neck, the tumor shrunk an inch and half. I am now able to sleep normally, no longer waking up from not being able to breathe, and my pills no longer get stuck. I am planning on being in full remission in a couple months!

The doctors gave me less than a year to live-that was six months ago! I can't wait to see the look on their faces when they see the tumors are shrinking! I get to prove them wrong; they told me there was no alternative care to cancer and that I was going to die. I haven't been this happy in years!!! I am no longer scared of my cancer! I cannot thank you enough, Elaine! Someday I hope to meet you in person and I would love for my kids to meet the person who helped save my life!

Kelly M. From California, USA

It's true, cancer doesn't scare me any more. After my diagnosis with Breast Cancer in 2009, I had a lumpectomy, but decided not to have radiotherapy and chemotherapy. A friend of mine had followed the alternative route with breast cancer, and her cancer returned destroying her health, and eventually taking her life; her last words to me were 'If I had my time over, I'd take everything the doctors offered, chemotherapy, radiotherapy, anything.'

Yet still when I got my diagnosis I knew that wasn't the right path for me. Elaine and I met online in 2010 when I was panicking after the discovery of 3 small new lumps – one in the original breast, and more worryingly, two in the other. Her dietary suggestions were added to my regimen and at my next scan, a month later, only one lump remained, and a month later there was nothing to see. I don't worry about cancer any more as I know that using the Cantin Ketogenic Diet I can suppress any recurrences. Elaine's information about allergies is so crucial for me as I already knew I was wheat and dairy intolerant, yet had let wheat slip back into my diet. I won't do that again.

Thank you Elaine for all your tireless efforts for all of us. You're a life-saver.

Gilli M. From London, U.K.

References

1. Hill, Lewis W., et al., *The Allen (Starvation) Treatment of Diabetes.* 4th ed. Boston: Leonard 1921. Print.
2. Freeman, John M., et al., *The Ketogenic Diet.* 4th ed. New York: DemosHealth 2007. Print. p.25-28
3. Hill, Lewis W., et al., *The Allen (Starvation) Treatment of Diabetes.* 4th ed. Boston: Leonard 1921. Print.
4. Evert A. *"Rethinking the Triad of Diabetes in the New Millennium."* ADA 20 Jun. 2009. Web. 18 May 2012.
    <http://spectrum.diabetesjournals.org/content/22/3/132.full>
5. *Joslin EP. A Diabetic Manual for the Mutual Use of Doctor and Patient. BiblioBazaarReproduction 2008. Print.*
6. Kossoff, Eric H., et al., *Ketogenic Diets.* 5th ed. New York: demosHEALTH 2011. Print. P.15-16.
7. Atkins, Robert C. *Dr.Atkins' Diet Revolution.* New York: Bantam Books 1973. Print.
8. Mayo Clinic. "Beta-Hydroxybutyrate, Serum". Mayo Medical Laboratories 1995. Web. 06 May 2012.
    <http://www.mayomedicallaboratories.com/test-catalog/print.php?unit_code=9251>
9. Jarrett, SG., et al. "The ketogenic diet increases mitochondrial glutathione levels." Online Library 04 May 2008. Web. 12 May 2012.
    <http://onlinelibrary.wiley.com/doi/10.1111/j.1471-4159.2008.05460.x/full>
10. Nagasawa, H. Personal interview. 26 Dec 2009.
    <http://www.youtube.com/watch?v=fYQibc32CfM>
11. Hyman, Mark. Personal interview. 18 Jul 2008.
    <http://www.youtube.com/watch?v=Eh2PYQBICWs>
12. Wikipedia. "Otto Heinrich Warburg". Wikipedia 10 May 2012. Web. 14 May 2012.
    <http://en.wikipedia.org/wiki/Otto_Heinrich_Warburg>
13. Moller, N, and J. Jorgensen. "Effects of Growth Hormone on Glucose, Lipid, and Protein Metabolism in Human Subjects." Endocrine Reviews April 2009. Web. 19 May 2012.
    <http://edrv.endojournals.org/content/30/2/152.full>

14. Langfort, J, et al. "Effect of low-carbohydrate-ketogenic diet on metabolic and hormonal responses to graded exercise in men." NCBI June 1996. Web. 19 May 2012.
<http://www.ncbi.nlm.nih.gov/pubmed/8807563>

15. Quigley, Max. " The Keto Diet For Women." .LiveStrong 29 Jul. 2011. Web. 19 May 2-12.
<http://www.livestrong.com/article/504942-the-keto-diet-for-women/>

16. Fine EJ, et al., "Acetoacetate reduces growth and ATP concentration in cancer cell lines which over-express uncoupling protein 2". The National Center for Biotechnology Information 29 May 2009. Web. 05 May 2012.
<http://www.ncbi.nlm.nih.gov/pubmed/19480693?ordinalpos=1&itool=EntrezSystem2.PEntrez.Pubmed.Pubmed_ResultsPanel.Pub>

17. Ross, Meyrizza. "Acetone in Children, children." Education and health-child. Jan 2010. Web. 05 May 2012.
<http://mikadokids.com/infant-and-child-health/acetone-in-children/>

18. Wikipedia. "Ketonuria." Wikipedia 25 Apr. 2012. Web. 5 May 2012.
<http://en.wikipedia.org/wiki/Ketonuria>

19. Nam-Seok, Joo, et al. " Ketonuria after Fasting may be Related to the Metabolic Superiority." NCBI Dec. 2010. 19 May 2012.
<http://www.ncbi.nlm.nih.gov/pmc/articles/PMC2995232/>

20. Jagatha, B, et al. "Curcumin treatment alleviates the effects of glutathione depletion in vitro and in vivo: therapeutic implications for Parkinson's disease explained via in silico studies." NCBI 1 March 2008. Web. 14 May 2012.
<http://www.ncbi.nlm.nih.gov/pubmed/18166164>

21. Santangelo, F. "Intracellular Thiol Concentration Modulating Inflammatory Response: Influence on the Regulation of Cell Functions Through Cysteine Prodrug Approach." Current Medicinal Chemistry, Volume 10, Number 23, December 2003 , pp. 2599-2610(12). Web. 12 May 2012.
<http://www.ingentaconnect.com/content/ben/cmc/2003/00000010/00000023/art00012>

22. Kumaran, VS., et al. "Repletion of antioxidant status by EGCG and retardation of oxidative damage induced macromolecular anomalies in aged rats." ScienceDirect 07 Nov 2007. Web 12 May 2012.
<http://www.sciencedirect.com/science/article/pii/S0531556507002495>

23. Crumley Hill S. "What Foods Increase Glutathione Levels?." LiveStrong 6 Nov 2009. Web 20 May 2012.
<http://www.livestrong.com/article/32331-foods-increase-glutathione-levels/>

24. Kuekids Australia. "Theoretical Basis Of The Ketogenic Diet." Kuekids Australia . Web. 12 May 2012.
<http://home.iprimus.com.au/kuekids/keto/kdbook/tbotkd.html>

25. Tisdale, MJ, et al. "Reduction of weight loss and tumour size in a cachexia model by a high fat diet." NCBI 1987 Jul;56(1):39-43. Web 12 May 2012.
<http://www.ncbi.nlm.nih.gov/pubmed/3620317>

26. Wang, Xiaobin, Pongracic JA, "Children's Memorial Food Allergy Study: Addressing major questions about food Allergies in children." Children's Memorial Hospital fall/winter 2009. Web. 10 May 2012.
<https://www.childrensmemorial.org/documents/research-fd_allergy_study-childsdocfall09.pdf>

27. Hill, Lewis W., et al., *The Allen (Starvation) Treatment of diabetes.* 4th ed. Boston: Leonard 1921. Print. P.8.

28. Freeman, John M., et al., *The Ketogenic Diet.* 4th ed. demosHEALTH 2007. Print.

29. Somers, Suzanne. *KNOCKOUT.* New York: Crown Publishers 2009. Print.

30. D'Adamo, Peter. "Eat right 4 Your Type." New York: Penguin Putnam 1996. Print.

31. O'Donohoe, PB, et al. "Exploring the clinical utility of blood ketone levels in the emergency department assessment of paediatric patients." EMJ 2006. Web. 20 May 2012.
<http://emj.bmj.com/content/23/10/783.abstract>

32. Wikipedia. "Ketonuria." Wikipedia 25 Apr. 2012. Web. 5 May 2012.
<http://en.wikipedia.org/wiki/Ketonuria>

33. Islets of Hope. "What Things Can Produce Ketones?" Islets of Hope 2006. Web. 19 May 2012. <http://www.isletsofhope.com/diabetes/care/ketones_1.html#produce>

34. Fife, Bruce. "Conquering Alzheimer's with Coconut Ketones." Coconut Research Center 2010. Web. 19 May 2012. <http://www.coconutresearchcenter.org/Conquering%20Alzheimers%20with%20Coconut%20Ketones.htm>

35. Lipsman, Mark. "What I learned from Cancer." GoodHealthInfo 2001. Web. 19 May 2012. <http://www.goodhealthinfo.net/cancer/what_i_learned.htm>

36. Pedersen, Dorothy. "Fasting Cured PH.D.'S Benign Jaw Tumor After Oncologist Told Her it Requires Surgery." Fasting Center International. Web 05 May 2012. < http://www.fasting.com/jawtumor.html>

37. Hoffard, Sammy. "Fasting-Healed of Ovarian Caner." Freedom You. Web. 12 May 2012. <http://www.freedomyou.com/fasting_book/healed_of_cancer.htm>

38. Wikipidia. "Otto Heinrich Warburg." Wikipidia 10 May 2012. Web 19 May 2012. < http://en.wikipedia.org/wiki/Otto_Heinrich_Warburg>

39. Heise, D. "Glucose: The Fuel of Cancer Cells". Heise Health Clinic 2011. Web. 19 May 2012. <http://www.drheise.com/cancersugar.htm>

40. MacArthur, J. "What is Lactic Acid?". WiseGEEK 2003. Web. 19 May 2012. <http://www.wisegeek.com/what-is-lactic-acid.htm>

41. Purac. "Lactic Acid". Lactic Acid. Web 22 May 2012. <http://www.lacticacid.com/lactic_acid_in_food.html>

42. Rofstad, E, et al. "Acidic extracellular pH promotes experimental metastasis of human melanoma cells in athymic nude mice." NCBI 2006. Web. 19 May 2012. <http://www.ncbi.nlm.nih.gov/pubmed/16818644>

43. Seyfried, TN, L. Sheldon, "Cancer as a Metabolic Disease". NCBI 2010. Web. 19 May 2012. <http://www.ncbi.nlm.nih.gov/pmc/articles/PMC2845135/>

44. Thuo, Joseph. "A New Hypothesis on Spontaneous Remission of Cancer". Second Opinions 02 Apr. 2010. Web. 04 May 2012
    <http://www.second-opinions.co.uk/thuo-hypothesis-2.html>.

45. MBVax. "William Coley". MBVax. Web. 13 May 2012.
    <http://www.mbvax.com/william_coley.htm>

46. MBVax. "Historical Results". MBVax. Web. 13 May 2012.
    <http://www.mbvax.com/historical_results.htm>

47. Martin, W. "Coley's Toxins: A Cancer Treatment History". Townsend Letter 2006. Web. 13 May 2012.
    <http://www.townsendletter.com/FebMar2006/coleystoxin0206.htm>

48. Cancer Research. "Our History." Cancer Research 2009. Web. 14 May 2012.
    <http://cancerresearch.org/history.html>

49. Rietz, D. "Dangers Of Milk And Dairy Products–The Facts". Rense.com 06 Jul. 2002. Web. 13 May 2012.
    <http://www.rense.com/general26/milk.htm>

50. Gandhi, M. "Milk & diabetes." Fairfield Life Mail Archive 29 Sept. 2005. Web. 13 May 2012.
    <http://www.mailarchive.com/fairfieldlife@yahoogroups.com/msg29997.html>

51. Schoffro Cook, M. "Harvard Declares Dairy NOT Part of a Healthy Diet." Care2 08 Jan 2012. Web. 14 May 2012.
    <http://www.care2.com/greenliving/harvard-declares-dairy-not-part-of-healthy-diet.html>

52. Food for Breast Cancer . "Milk is not recommended for breast cancer". Food for Breast Cancer. Web. 13 May 2012.
    <http://foodforbreastcancer.com/foods/milk>

53. Plant, Jane. "Cure Breast Cancer by Avoiding All Milk Products". AlkalizeForHealth 24 Jan 2000. Web. 13 May 2012.
    <http://www.alkalizeforhealth.net/Lnotmilk6.htm>

54. Plimpton, G. "Not Milk". NotMilk.com. Web. 13 May 2012.
    <http://www.notmilk.com/>

55. Cowen, Robert. "No Milk: D is for Diabetes". AFH 11 Dec. 2000. Web. 13 May 2012.
    <http://www.alkalizeforhealth.net/Lnotmilk10.htm>

56. Lane, WM, et al. "The Use of Cow's Milk in infancy". Pediatrics 91 (1993). Web. 21 May 2012.
<http://pediatrics.aappublications.org/content/91/2/515.2.abstract>

57. Cohen, R. "Multiple Sclerosis and the Dairy Link." Dairy Truth 2006. Web. 19 May 2012.
<http://www.dairytruth.com/2006/09/>

58. Cohen R. "Say No Way! To Whey!." Dairy Truth 2006. Web. 19 May 2012.
<http://www.dairytruth.com/2006/08/22/say-no-way-to-whey/>

59. "Dairy and Diabetes". Personal Interview 2010
<http://www.youtube.com/watch?v=j8FNaOYAJOM>

60. "Monsanto Cancer Milk." Wilson, S and J, Akre Investigative Documentary Video.
<http://www.youtube.com/watch?v=gVKvzHWuJRU>

61. Gerson.Org. "Foods For The Gerson Diet". Gerson.org. Web. 12 May 2012.
<http://gerson.org/pdfs/Foods_For_The_Gerson_Diet.pdf>

62. Klotter, Jule. "Film Documents Cancer 'Warriors' Survival." FindArticles 2010. Web. 12 May 2012.
<http://findarticles.com/p/articles/mi_7396/is_325-326/ai_n55187949/>

63. Thurnell-Read, J. "What Is The Gerson Therapy?." Healthandgoodness 2012. Web 14 May 2012.
<http://www.healthandgoodness.com/article/gerson-therapy-information.html>

64. Hildenbrand, G., andMora, A. "Overview of immunotherapy treatments". Gar Hildenbrand July 2011. Web. 05 May2012.
<http://garhildenbrand.com/overview.html>

65. Mercola, J. "A Special Interview with Dr. Nicholas Gonzalez by: Dr. Mercola". Mercola.com 23 Apr. 2011. Web. 11 May 2011.
<http://mercola.fileburst.com/PDF/ExpertInterviewTranscripts/Interview-Gonzalez-on-Alternative-Cancer-Treatments.pdf>

66. Kuekids Australia. "Theoretical Basis Of The Ketogenic Diet". Kuekids Australia . Web. 12 May 2012.

<http://home.iprimus.com.au/kuekids/keto/kdbook/tbot kd.html>

67. Kossoff, Eric H., et al., *Ketogenic Diets.* 5th ed. New York: demosHEALTH 2011. Print. p. 35 and p 61.

68. Coussens, L, and Z. Werb. "Inflammatory Cells and Cancer". NCBI March 2001. Web. 19 May 2012.
<http://www.ncbi.nlm.nih.gov/pmc/articles/PMC21934 19/>

69. Eliaz, Isaac. "Help Your Body Win The Battle Against Autoimmune Disease". Easy Health Options 11 Dec 2011. Web. 03 Jan 2012.
<http://www.easyhealthoptions.com/alternative-medicine/help-your-body-win-the-battle-against-autoimmune-disease/>

70. Lee SK, et al. "Vitamin C suppresses proliferation of the human melanoma cell SK-MEL-2 through the inhibition of cyclooxygenase-2 (COX-2) expression and the modulation of insulin-like growth factor II (IGF-II) production." NCBI JUL 2008. Web. 16 May 2012
<http://www.ncbi.nlm.nih.gov/pubmed/18297687>

71. MedicineNet. "Definition of COX-2". MedicineNet 19 March 2012. Web. 23 May 2012.
<http://www.medterms.com/script/main/art.asp?articl ekey=7121>

72. O'Leary KA, et al. "Effect of flavonoids and vitamin E on cyclooxygenase-2 (COX-2) transcription." NCBI 13 JUL 2004. Web. 16 May 2012.
<http://www.ncbi.nlm.nih.gov/pubmed/15225597>

73. Goel, A, et al., "Specific inhibition of cyclooxygenase-2 (COX-2) expression by dietary curcumin in HT-29 human colon cancer cells." NCBI 30 OCT 2001. Web. 16 May 2012.
<http://www.ncbi.nlm.nih.gov/pubmed/11566484>

74. Chen CH, et al. "Suppression of endotoxin-induced proinflammatory responses by citrus pectin through blocking LPS signaling pathways." NCBI OCT 2006. Web. 16 May 2012.
<http://www.ncbi.nlm.nih.gov/pubmed/16930561>

75. Zykova TA, et al. "Resveratrol Directly Targets COX-2 to Inhibit Carcinogenesis". NCBI OCT 2008. Web. 16 May 2012.
<http://www.ncbi.nlm.nih.gov/pmc/articles/PMC2562941/>

76. Gibellini, L. Et al. "Interfering with ROS Metabolism in Cancer Cells: The Potential Role of Quercetin". MDPI 14 Jun 2012. Web. 13 May 2012.
<http://www.mdpi.com/2072-6694/2/2/1288>

77. Velmurugan B, et al. "Dietary feeding of grape seed extract prevents intestinal tumorigenesis in APCmin/+ mice." NCBI Jan. 2010. Web. 16 May 2012.
< http://www.ncbi.nlm.nih.gov/pubmed/20072658>

78. Harzenberg, LA, et al. "Glutathione deficiency is associated with impaired survival in HIV disease". PNAS 1997. Web. 15 May.
<http://www.pnas.org/content/94/5/1967.full>

79. English, J, and W. Dean. "Citrus Pectin". Nutrition Review 2011. Web. 22 May 2012.
<http://www.nutritionreview.org/library/citrus.pectin.php>

80. Perez-Guisado, J., et al. "Spanish Ketogenic Mediterranean diet: a healthy cardiovascular diet for weight loss". Nutrition Journal 2008, 7:30 doi:10.1186/1475- 891-7-30
<http://www.nutritionj.com/content/7/1/30>

81. Chan, A. " Low Carb, high-fat diet could replace dialysis". MSNBC 20 Apr. 2011. Web. 14 May 2012.
<http://www.msnbc.msn.com/id/42689095/ns/health/t/low-carb-High-fat-diet-could-replace-dialysis/>

82. Fiore, K. "Supplement Averts kidney Stones in Ketogenic Diet". Medpage Today 22 Jul 2009. Web. 16 May 2012.
<http://www.medpagetoday.com/Nephrology/GeneralNephrology/15204>

83. Barclay, L. "Oral Potassium Citrate May Help Prevent Kidney Stones in Children on the Ketogenic Diet". Medscape 27 Jul 2009. Web. 16 May 2012.
<http://www.medscape.com/viewarticle/706503>

84. Wikipedia. "Acetone". Wikipedia 14 May 2012. Web. 16 May 2012.
<http://en.wikipedia.org/wiki/Acetone>

85. Campbell. "How I beat cancer". Green Drinks Diaries Oct 2011. Web. 16 May 2012.
<http://www.greendrinkdiaries.com/how-i-beat-cancer/>

86. Laino, C. "Pregnancy Hormone May Prevent Breast Cancer". FoxNews 20 Apr. 2005. Web. 23 May 2012.
<http://www.foxnews.com/story/0,2933,153964,00.html>

87. Gauthier T, et al. "Respiration of mitochondria isolated from differentiated and undifferentiated HT29 colon cancer cells in the presence of various substrates and ADP generating systems". ScienceDirect 2002. Web. 23 May 2012.
<http://www.sciencedirect.com/science/article/pii/0020711X9090145S>

88. Allan, Christian B., and Wolfgang Lutz. *Life Without Bread.* Los Angeles: Keats Publishing 2000. Print. P. 169.

89. Wigmore, Ann. "Dr. Ann Wigmore's Life Story Raw Living Foods 20 May 2010. Web. 14 May 2012.
<http://rawlivingfoods.typepad.com/1/2010/05/dr-ann-wigmores-life-story.html>

90. Allan, Christian B., and Wolfgang Lutz. *Life Without Bread.* Los Angeles: Keats Publishing 2000. Print. P. 1-3.

91. Virgin Coconut Oil. ""Virgin Coconut Oil "Miracle Cure for Cancer""Virgin Coconut Oil 2010. Web. 26 May 2012.
<http://www.thevirgincoconutoil.com/articleitem.php?articleid=176>

92. Chow, R. "Anti-Cancer Properties of Olives Revealed in Two Recent Studies". NaturalNews 11 Feb. 2009. Web. 26 May 2012.
<http://www.naturalnews.com/025593_cancer_natural_olives.html>

93. The Beautiful Truth". Krocshel, Steve. 2008. Documentary. <http://articles.mercola.com/sites/articles/archive/2011/08/14/beautiful-truth-about-outlawed-cancer-treatment.aspx?e_cid=20110814_SNL_Art_1>

94. Moser, IA. "Healing Testimony: Terminal Breast Cancer". Healing Cancer Naturally Nov 2008. Web. 12 May 2012. <http://www.healingcancernaturally.com/terminal-breastcure-wheatgrass.html>

95. Toronto Radio Interview. "Interview with Dr. med. Ryke Geerd Hamer". Healing Cancer Naturally 13 March 1999. Web. 13 May 2012. <http://www.healingcancernaturally.com/hamer6.html#interview-with-dr-ryke-geerd-hamer-md>

96. Somers, Suzanne. *KNOCKOUT*. New York: Crown Publishers 2009. Print.

97. Freeman, John M., et al., *The Ketogenic Diet*. 4ᵗʰ ed. demosHEALTH 2007. Print. p. 40.

98. Mercola J. "Warning: This Daily Habit is Damaging Your Bones, Brain, Kidneys, and Thyroid". Mercola.com Jul. 2010. Web. 27 May 2012 <http://articles.mercola.com/sites/articles/archive/2010/07/01/paul-connett-interview.aspx>

99. Mercola J. "Tap Water Toxins: Is Your Water Trying to Kill You?". Mercola.com Feb 2009. Web. 27 May 2012. <http://articles.mercola.com/sites/articles/archive/2009/02/05/tap-water-toxins-is-your-water-trying-to-kill-you.aspx>

100. Curezone. "Fluoride and Aluminum - toxic combination of fluoroaluminum complex". Curezone. Web 27 May 2012. <http://curezone.com/art/read.asp?ID=11&db=12&C0=12>

101. Forbes WF and DR McLachlan. "Further thoughts on the aluminum-Alzheimer's disease link." NCBI Aug. 1996. Web. 27 May 2012. <http://www.ncbi.nlm.nih.gov/pubmed/8882222>

102. Fluoride Action Network. "HEALTH EFFECTS: Fluoride & the Brain". Fluoride Action Network 2007. Web. 27 May 2012. <http://www.fluoridealert.org/health/brain/>

103. The Beautiful Truth". Krocshel, Steve. 2008. Documentary Movie. <http://articles.mercola.com/sites/articles/archive/2011/08/14/beautiful-truth-about-outlawed-cancer-treatment.aspx?e_cid=20110814_SNL_Art_1>

104. Yiamouyiannis, John. "Fluoride The Silent Killer". Consumer Health Jan. 1998. Web. 27 May 2012. <http://www.consumerhealth.org/articles/display.cfm?ID=19990303222823>

105. Maugh II, T. "Research shows promise in reversing Type 1 diabetes". LA Times 25 Jun 2011. Web. 12 May 2012. <http://articles.latimes.com/2011/jun/25/health/la-he-bcg-diabetes-20110625>

106. BroadviewCare. "Acetone in Children". BroadviewCare June 2009. Web 22 May 2012. <http://www.broadviewcare.org/acetona_ninos.php>

107. Wikipedia. "Sickness Behaviour". Wikipedia 12 May 2012. Web. 26 May 2012. <http://en.wikipedia.org/wiki/Sickness_behavior>

108. Thuo, Joseph. "A New Hypothesis on Spontaneous Remission of Cancer". Second Opinions 02 Apr. 2010. Web. 04 May 2012. <http://www.second-opinions.co.uk/thuo-hypothesis-2.html>.

109. Mercola, J. "A Special Interview with Dr. Nicholas Gonzalez by: Dr. Mercola". Mercola.com 23 Apr. 2011. Web. 11 May 2011. <http://mercola.fileburst.com/PDF/ExpertInterviewTranscripts/Interview-Gonzalez-on-Alternative-Cancer-Treatments.pdf>

110. Cooper, Thea, and Arthur Ainsberg. *BREAKTHROUGH*. New York: St. Martin's Press 2010. Print.

111. Virgin Coconut Oil. ""Virgin Coconut Oil "Miracle Cure for Cancer""Virgin Coconut Oil 2010. Web. 26 May 2012. <http://www.thevirgincoconutoil.com/articleitem.php?articleid=176>

112. Minton, BL. "New Study Finds Olive Oil Effective against HER-2 Breast Cancer". NaturalNews 11 Jan. 2009. Web. 26 May 2012. <http://www.naturalnews.com/025290_oil_olive_fat.html>

113. "Coconut Oil Ketones Increase Blood Circulation to Brain". Mary Newport. Personal interview <http://alzheimersweekly.com/content/coconut-oil-ketones-increase-blood-circulation-brain>

114. Veech RL, et al. "" A ketone ester diet increases brain malonyl-CoA and Uncoupling proteins 4 and 5 while decreasing food intake in the normal Wistar Rat." NCBI Aug. 2010. Web. 27 May 2012.

115. Coconut Oil Ketones Increase Blood Circulation to Brain". Mary Newport. Personal interview <http://alzheimersweekly.com/content/coconut-oil-ketones-increase-blood-circulation-brain>

116. Kossoff, Eric H., et al., *Ketogenic Diets.* 5th ed. New York: demosHEALTH 2011. Print. P. 281.

ELAINE CANTIN

REFERENCES GROUPED BY SUBJECT

DIETS, HERBS & SUPPLEMENTS

Freeman, John M., et al., *The Ketogenic Diet*. 4th ed.demosHEALTH 2007. Print.

Kossoff, Eric H., et al., *Ketogenic Diets*. 5th ed. New York: demosHEALTH 2011. Print.

Somers, Suzanne. *KNOCKOUT*. New York: Crown Publishers 2009. Print.

Cooper, Thea, and Arthur Ainsberg. *BREAKTHROUGH*. New York: St. Martin's Press 2010. Print.

Sisson, Mark. *The Primal Blueprint*. Malibu: Primal Nutrition 2009. Print.

Hill, Lewis W., et al., *The Allen (starvation) treatment of diabetes*. 4th ed. Boston: Leonard 1921. Print.

Allan, Christian B., and Wolfgang Lutz. *Life Without Bread.* Los Angeles: Keats Publishing 2000. Print.

Atkins, Robert C. *Dr. Atkin's' Diet Revolution.* York: Bantam Books 1973. Print.

D'Adamo, Peter. "Eat right 4 Your Type." New
        York: Penguin Putnam 1996. Print.

Reuters. "First of its Kind Botanical Formula Shows
        Promise for Incurable Breast Cancer." Reuters.
        01 Aug. 2012. Web. 01 Aug 2012.
<http://www.reuters.com/article/2012/08/01/idUS1160
21+01-Aug-2012+PRN20120801>

CANCER, KETONES & SUGAR

Wikipedia. "Otto Heinrich Warburg". Wikipedia
        10 May 2012. Web. 14 May 2012.
<http://en.wikipedia.org/wiki/Otto_Heinrich_Warburg>

Webb Hill, L, and RS Heckman. "The Allen
        (starvation) treatment of diabetes". Google
        2012. Web. 14 May 2012.
<http://books.google.com/books?id=aYQPAAAAYAA
J&printsec=frontcover&source=gbs_ge_summary_r&c
ad=0#v=onepage&q&f=false>

Thuo, Joseph. "A New Hypothesis on Spontaneous
        Remission of Cancer". Second Opinions 02
        Apr. 2010. Web. 04 May 2012.
 <http://www.second-opinions.co.uk/thuo-hypothesis-
2.html>.

Fine EJ, et al., "Acetoacetate reduces growth and ATP
        concentration in cancer cell lines which over-
        express uncoupling protein 2". The National
        Center for Biotechnology Information 29 May 2009.
        Web. 05 May 2012.
<http://www.ncbi.nlm.nih.gov/pubmed/19480693?ordi
nalpos=1&itool=EntrezSystem2.PEntrez.Pubmed.Pubm
ed_ResultsPanel.Pub>

ELAINE CANTIN

Unknown. "Acetone in children". WIKI NOTICIA 02
    NOV. 2010. Web. 05 MAY 2012.
<http://en.wikinoticia.com/lifestyle/Maternity/64309-
acetone-in-children>

Ross, Meyrizza. "Acetone, Acetone in Children,
    children, Increased fever, symptom of disease".
    Education, Maternal   and child health Jan 2010.
    Web. 05 May 2012.
<http://mikadokids.com/infant-and-child-
health/acetone-in-children/>

Habeck, Michael. "Acetone". Eco-usa.net May 1994.
    Web. 05 May 2012.
<http://www.ecousa.net/toxics/chemicals/acetone.shtml
>

Sisson, Mark. "A Primal Primer: Leptin". Marks' Daily
    Apple17 Jun. 2011. Web. 06 May 2012.
<http://www.marksdailyapple.com/leptin/#axzz1gjN
RET5K>

Brandt, M. "The Synthesis and Utilization of Ketone
    Bodies". Rose-Hulman Institute 2000. Web
    May 19 2012.
<http://www.rose-
hulman.edu/~brandt/Chem330/Ketone_bodies.pdf>

Unknown. "Definition of Alkalosis". MedicineNet.com
    19 Mar. 2012. Web. 06 May 2012.
<http://www.medterms.com/script/main/art.asp?articlekey
=6852>

Dugdale, David C. "Alkalosis". AARP 15 Nov. 2009.
        Web. 06 May 2012.
<http://healthtools.aarp.org/adamcontent/alkalosis?CMP=
KNC-360I-GOOGLE-
HEA&HBX_PK=alkalosis&utm_source=Google&utm_m
edium=cpc&utm_term=alkalosis&utm_campaign=G_Dise
ases%2Band%2BConditions&360cid=SI_148896666_649
5451981_1>

RMALaboratory. "Food Allergy in the news". Rocky
        Mountain Analytical 2007. Web. 06 May 2012.
<http://www.rmalab.com/index.php?id=18>

Wikipidia. "Adenosine Triphosphate". Wikipidia 28
        Apr. 2012. Web. 06 May 2012.
<http://en.wikipedia.org/wiki/Adenosine_triphosphate

3 KETONE BODY SOURCES

Mayo Clinic. "Beta-Hydroxybutyrate, Serum". Mayo
        Medical Laboratories 1995. Web. 06 May 2012.
<http://www.mayomedicallaboratories.com/test-
catalog/print.php?unit_code=9251>

Rattue, Petra. "Breast Cancer Prevention - Part Time
        Low Carb Diet Better Than Standard Full Time
        Diets". Medical News
        Today 10 Dec. 2011. Web. 06 May 2012.
 <http://www.medicalnewstoday.com/articles/23899
1.php>

Wang, Xiaobin, Pongracic JA, "Children's Memorial
    Food Allergy Study: Addressing major questions
    about food Allergies in children". Children's
    Memorial Hospital fall/winter 2009. Web. 10
    May 2012.
<https://www.childrensmemorial.org/documents/resear
ch-fd_allergy_study-childsdocfall09.pdf>

**ALZHEIMER DISEASE, OTHER DISORDERS &
KETONES**

"Coconut Oil Ketones Increase Blood Circulation to
    Brain". Mary Newport. Personal interview
<http://alzheimersweekly.com/content/coconut-oil-
ketones-increase-blood-circulation-brain>

Dobromylskyj P, "Alzheimers and Ketone". High-Fat-
    Nutrition Dec. 2008. Web. 27 May 2012.
<http://high-fat-
nutrition.blogspot.com/2008/12/alzheimers-and-
ketones.html>

Veech RL. "The therapeutic implications of ketone
    bodies: the effects of ketone bodies in
    pathological conditions: ketosis, ketogenic diet,
    redox states, insulin resistance, and
    mitochondrial metabolism." NCBI March 2004.
    Web 27 May 2012.
<http://www.ncbi.nlm.nih.gov/pubmed/14769489>

Masino SA, et al. "Adenosine, Ketogenic Diet and
    Epilepsy: The Emerging Therapeutic
    Relationship Between Metabolism and Brain
    Activity". NCBI Sept. 2009. Web 27 May 2012.
<http://www.ncbi.nlm.nih.gov/pmc/articles/PMC27690
09/>

RELATION BETWEEN KETONE & HORMONES

Alberti KG, et al. "Hormonal regulation of ketone-
body metabolism in man." NCBI 1978. Web. 19
May 2012.
<http://www.ncbi.nlm.nih.gov/pubmed/749914>

Moller, N, and J. Jorgensen. "Effects of Growth
Hormone onGlucose, Lipid, and Protein
Metabolism in Human Subjects". Endocrine
Reviews April 2009. Web. 19 May 2012.
<http://edrv.endojournals.org/content/30/2/152.full>

The American Medical Heritage Dictionary
"Compensated
Acidosis" The free Dictionary 2007. Web. 12 May
2012.
<http://medical-
dictionary.thefreedictionary.com/compensated+acidosis>

Fife, Bruce. "Conquering Alzheimer's with Coconut
Ketones". Coconut Research Center 2010. Web.
12 May 2012.
<http://www.coconutresearchcenter.org/Conquering%20Alzheimer
s%20with%20Coconut%20Ketones.htm>

rBGH

"Monsanto Cancer Milk". Wilson, S and Akre J. Investigative
Documentary Video.
<http://www.youtube.com/watch?v=gVKvzHWuJRU>

ACS. "Recombinant Bovine Growth Hormone". ACS
18 Feb. 2011. Web. 27 May 2012.
<http://www.cancer.org/Cancer/CancerCauses/OtherCa
rcinogens/AtHome/recombinant-bovine-growth-
hormone>

FASTING

The Nazarene Way. "Fasting". MCTV 14 Jan 2012.
    Web 05 May 2012.
<http://www.mychristiantv.net/health/fasting/81606987
.html>

Pederson, Dorothy. "FASTING CURED PH.D.'S
    BENIGN JAW TUMOR AFTER
    ONCOLOGIST TOLD HER IT
    EQUIRES SURGERY". Fasting Center
    International. Web 05 May 2012.
< http://www.fasting.com/jawtumor.html>

Hoffard, Sammy. "Fasting-Healed of Ovarian Caner".
    Freedom You. Web. 12 May 2012.
<http://www.freedomyou.com/fasting_book/healed_of_
cancer.htm>

KETOGENIC DIET

Caveman2.0. "Intermittent Fasting Part Two-
    Hormones, tissue repair and your brain".
    Caveman2.0 18 Apr. 2010. Web.05 May 2012.
    <http://caveman2point0.blogspot.com/2010/04/i
    ntermittent-fasting-part-two-hormones.html>

Friebe, Richard. "Can a High-Fat Diet Beat Cancer?"
    Time Health 17 Sept. 2007. Web. 06 May 2012.
<http://www.time.com/time/health/article/0,8599,16624
84,00.html>

Nebeling LC, et al. "Effects of a ketogenic diet on
        tumor metabolism and nutritional status in
        pediatric oncology patients: two case reports."
        Apr;14(2):202-8. Web 12 May 2012.
<http://www.ncbi.nlm.nih.gov/sites/entrez?cmd=Retrie
ve&db=PubMed&list_uids=7790697&dopt=AbstractPl
us&holding=f1000%2Cf1000m%2Cisrctn>

Tisdale, MJ, et al. "Reduction of weight loss and
        tumour size in a cachexia model by a high fat
        diet." Br J Cancer. 1987 Jul;56(1):39-43. Web
        12 May 2012.
<http://www.ncbi.nlm.nih.gov/pubmed/3620317>

Standford U Med Center"Ketogenic Diet Meal
        Planner". Stanford University 23 Jan 2006.
Web. 12 May 2012..
<http://www.stanford.edu/group/ketodiet/>

Cox, CL. "Ketogenic Diet and Cancer - Diet as a
        Cancer Solution". CancerSolutions.Org. 14
        Sept. 2009. Web.12 May 2012.
<http://www.cancersolutions.org/2009/09/ketogenic-
diet-and-cancer-diet-as.html>

Emory University. "Ketogenic Diet Prevents Seizures
        ByEnhancing Brain Energy Production,
        Increasing Neuron Stability" Emory University
        14 Nov 2005. Web. May 12 2012.
<http://www.whsc.emory.edu/press_releases2.cfm?ann
ouncement_id_seq=5179>

Seyfried, Tn, Mukherjee, P. "Targeting energy
        metabolism in brain cancer: review and hypothesis".
        Nutrition&Metabolism 2005. Web. 12 May 2012.
<http://www.nutritionandmetabolism.com/content/2/1/3
0>

Wikipedia. "Ketonuria". Wikipedia 25 Apr. 2012.
        Web. 5 May 2012.
<http://en.wikipedia.org/wiki/Ketonuria>

Parker, Steve. "Recommended Supplements for the
        Ketogenic Mediterranean Diet". Diabetic
        Mediterranean Diet 01 Nov. 2009. Web. 05 May
        2012.
<http://diabeticmediterraneandiet.com/2009/11/01/reco
mmended-supplements-for-the-ketogenic-
mediterranean-diet/>

Ketogenic Diet Resource. "Ketosis: Survival over
        Starvation". Ketogenic Diet Resource 2011.
        Web. 12 May 2012.
<http://www.ketogenic-diet-resource.com/ketosis.html>

Zuccoli , et al. "Metabolic management of
        glioblastoma multiforme using standard therapy
        together with restricted
        ketogenic diet: Case Report".
        Nutrition&Metabolism 22 Apr. 2010. Web. 12
        May 2012.
<http://www.nutritionandmetabolism.com/content/7/1/3
3>

AlphaGalileo Foundation. "Oestrogen Reduces
        Aggression In Breast Cancer". MNT 15 Feb
        2011. Web. 12 May 2012.
<http://www.medicalnewstoday.com/articles/216450.ph
p>

Kuekids Australia. "Theoretical Basis Of The
        Ketogenic Diet". Kuekids Australia . Web. 12
        May 2012.
<http://home.iprimus.com.au/kuekids/keto/kdbook/
tbotkd.html>

Zhou, W., et al. "The calorically restricted ketogenic diet, an effective alternative therapy for malignant brain cancer". NCBI 21 Feb 2007. Web. 12 May 2012.
<http://www.ncbi.nlm.nih.gov/pmc/articles/PMC1819381/>

KETONE BODIES

Wikipedia. "Ketone Bodies". Wikipedia 24 May 2012. Web. 26 May 2012.
<http://en.wikipedia.org/wiki/Ketone_bodies>

ACETONE & FEVER

Wikipedia. "Fever". Wikipedia 25 May 2012. Web. 26 May 2012.
< http://en.wikipedia.org/wiki/Fever>

Wikipedia. "Sickness Behaviour". Wikipedia 12 May 2012. Web. 26 May 2012.
<http://en.wikipedia.org/wiki/Sickness_behavior>

GERSON AND COLEY'S TOXINS

Gerson.Org. "Foods For The Gerson Diet". Gerson.org. Web. 12 May 2012.
<http://gerson.org/pdfs/Foods_For_The_Gerson_Diet.pdf>

Klotter, Jule. "Film Documents Cancer 'Warriors' Survival". FindArticles 2010. Web. 12 May 2012.
 <http://findarticles.com/p/articles/mi_7396/is_325-326/ai_n55187949/>

Thurnell-Read, J. "What Is The Gerson Therapy?". Healthandgoodness 2012. Web 14 May 2012.
<http://www.healthandgoodness.com/article/gerson-therapy-information.html>

REVERSING TYPE I DIABETES

Maugh II, T. "Research shows promise in reversing Type 1 diabetes". LA Times 25 Jun 2011. Web. 12 May 2012.
<http://articles.latimes.com/2011/jun/25/health/la-he-bcg-diabetes-20110625>

HIGHER RISK OF GETTING BREAST CANCER IF YOU HAVE TYPE 2 DIABETES

Schrauder, MJ, et al. "Diabetes and prognosis in a breast cancer cohort." NCBI. Jun. 2011. Web. 20 May 2012.
<http://www.ncbi.nlm.nih.gov/pubmed/21132511>

SUGAR/FRUCTOSE CANCER

Heise Health Clinic. "The Cancer-Sugar Connection". Heise Healt Clinic 2011. Web. 12 May 2012.
<http://www.drheise.com/cancersugar.htm>

JP. "The Prostate Cancer Diet". Healthy Fellow 29
        May 2009. Web. 12 May 2012.
<http://www.healthyfellow.com/249/the-prostate-
cancer-diet/>

Bollig-Fischer, A, et al. "Oncogene activation induces
        metabolic transformation resulting in insulin-
        independence in human breast cancer cells".
        NCBI March 2011. Web. 26 May 2012.
<http://www.ncbi.nlm.nih.gov/pubmed/21437235>

NewTreatments.org. "Tumors decrease in size when a
        person stops eating carbohydrates". New
        Treatments 2003. Web. 12 May 2012.
<http://www.newtreatments.org/cancer>

Zhang, X., et al. "Tumor pH and Its Measurement".
        JNM 2010. Web. 12 May 2012.
<http://jnm.snmjournals.org/content/51/8/1167.full>

Mercola J. "Startling NEW Evidence: This Drink
        Causes Your Neurons to Stagnate for 20
        Minutes". Mercola.com Feb. 2011. Web. 27
        May 2012.
<http://articles.mercola.com/sites/articles/archive/2011/
02/28/new-study-confirms-fructose-affects-your-brain-
very-differently-than-glucose.aspx>

Appleton N. "Fructose is No Answer for a
        Sweetener". Mercola.com Jan. 2002. Web. 27
        May 2012.
<http://articles.mercola.com/sites/articles/archive/2002/
01/05/fructose-part-two.aspx>

Wikia. "Type I Diabetes". Wikia. Web. 05 May 2012.
 <http://diabetes.wikia.com/wiki/Type_1_diabetes>

Freeman, JM. "What every pediatrician should know about the ketogenic diet". Curezone.com 21 Nov. 2004. Web. 1 May 2012.
<http://curezone.com/forums/fm.asp?i=56036>

Wheless, JW. "History and Origin of the Ketogenic Diet". Online Library 4 Nov 2008. Web. 13 May 2012.
<http://onlinelibrary.wiley.com/doi/10.1111/j.1528-1167.2008.01821.x/full>

FOOD AND SUPPLEMENTS WITH ANTI_CANCER PROPERTIES
(kelp, red clover, watercress, olives, coconut oil, iodine, chlorella, Spirulina, graviola, turmeric, melatonin, kale, coriander, ginger, garlic, rosemary

A.R.E. "Renee Caisse's Herbal Tea". Edgar Cayce. Web 26 May 2012.
<http://www.edgarcaycehouston.org/Research.htm>

Wikipedia. "Chlorella". Wikipedia 8 May 2012. Web. 26 May 2012.
<http://en.wikipedia.org/wiki/Chlorella>

Adams, M. "Vitamin A produces astonishing leukemia cure rate, even without chemotherapy". NaturalNews 10 Jun. 2004. Web. 26 May 2012.
<http://www.naturalnews.com/001123_cancer_chemotherapy.html>

Baliga, MS and S. Rao. "Radioprotective potential of mint: A brief review". Cancer Journal 2012. Web. 26 May 2012.
<http://www.cancerjournal.net/article.asp?issn=0973-1482;year=2010;volume=6;issue=3;spage=255;epage=262;aulast=Baliga>

HealthDiaries. "20 Health Benefits of Turmeric". HealthDiaries Oct 2007. Web 26 May 2012.
<http://www.healthdiaries.com/eatthis/20-health-benefits-of-turmeric.html>

English, J. and D. Ward. "modified Citrus Pectin Inhibition of Cancer Cells growth and Metastases". Nutrition Review 2011. Web. 26 May 2012.
<http://www.nutritionreview.org/library/citrus.pectin.php>

UMMC. "Melatonin". U of Maryland Jan. 2012. Web. 26 May 2012.
<http://www.umm.edu/altmed/articles/melatonin-000315.htm>

University of Haifa Israel. "Sleep in a darkened room to reduce your chances of cancer". WDDTY 8 Sept. 2010. Web. 26 May 2012.
<http://www.wddty.com/sleep-in-a-darkened-room-to-reduce-your-chances-of-cancer.html>

Walker, S. "How Can Adding Lemon Juice to Water Make the Water Alkaline?". eHow. Web. 26 May 2012.
<http://www.ehow.com/about_5373187_can-water-make-water-alkaline.html>

Whfoods. "Kale". Whfoods. Web. 26 May 2012.
<http://www.whfoods.com/genpage.php?tname=foodsp
ice&dbid=38>

Williams D. "Cilantro Chelation - That Can Save
        Your Life". NewsMediaExplorer Feb. 2006.
        Web. 26 May 2012.
<http://www.newmediaexplorer.org/chris/2006/02/19/ci
lantro_chelation_that_can_save_your_life.htm>

Bker, L. "Breast cancer breakthrough: watercress turns
        off signal that causes tumors to develop".
        NaturalNews 13 Oct. 2010. Web. 26 May 2012.
<http://www.naturalnews.com/030029_watercress_tum
ors.html>

Kowalska, E, et al. "Increased rates of chromosome
        Breakage in BRCA1 carriers are normalized by oral
        selenium supplementation". NCBI May 2005. Web.
        26 May 2012.
<http://www.ncbi.nlm.nih.gov/pubmed?term=Increased
%20rates%20of%20chromosome%20breakage%20in%
20BRCA1%20carriers%20are%20normalized%20by%
20oral%20selenium%20supplementation.>

Pierce, RM. "Cleanse & Alkalize Naturally with
        Lemon & Aloe Vera". 09 Aug. 2010. Web. 26
        may 2012.
<http://www.naturesfare.com/blog/vitamins/cleanse-
alkalize-naturally-with-lemons-aloe-vera/>

Venturi, S, et al. "Role of iodine in evolution and
        carcinogenesis of thyroid, breast and stomach".
        Ithyroid Jan. 2000. Web. 26 May 2012.
< http://www.ithyroid.com/cancer.htm>

Cancer Cure Foundation"Cancer Fighting Foods/Spices". CanCure.org. Web. 26 May 2012.
<http://www.cancure.org/cancer_fighting_foods.htm>

COLEY

Wikipedia. "Coley's Toxins". Wikipedia 27 Apr. 2012, Web. 13 May 2012.
<http://en.wikipedia.org/wiki/Coley_Vaccine>

MBVax. "William Coley". MBVax. Web. 13 May 2012.
<http://www.mbvax.com/william_coley.htm>

MBVax. "Historical Results". MBVax. Web. 13 May 2012.
<http://www.mbvax.com/historical_results.htm>

Martin, W. "Coley's Toxins: A Cancer Treatment History". Townsend Letter 2006. Web. 13 May 2012.
<http://www.townsendletter.com/FebMar2006/coleysto xin0206.htm>

Cancer Research. "Our History". Cancer Research 2009. Web. 14 May 2012.
<http://cancerresearch.org/history.html>

Moss, RW. "Microbially induced fever and spontaneous cancer remissions ("Coley's toxins")". Healing cancer naturally Sept. 2002. Web. 20 march 2012.
<http://healingcancernaturally.com/nature_heals2.html# Coley's_toxins>

Thuo, Joseph. "A New Hypothesis on Spontaneous
       Remission of Cancer". Damar Institute
       unknown date. Web. 15 March 2012.
<http://damarinstitute.ca/cancerremission.html>

Narkia Natti. "Coley'sToxins / Issel's Fever Therapy".
       Cancer Guide. 19 Apr. 1996. Web. 15 March
       2012.
<http://cancerguide.org/coley.html>

MD Anderson Cancer Center. "Coley Toxins Detailed
       Scientific Review". University Of Texas MD
       Anderson Cancer Center . Web. 15 March 2012.
<http://www.mdanderson.org/education-and-
research/resources-for-professionals/clinical-tools-and-
resources/cimer/therapies/nonplant-biologic-organic-
pharmacologic-therapies/coley-toxins-scientific.html>

Hildenbrand, G., and Mora, A. "Overview of
       Immunotherapy treatments". Gar Hildenbrand
       July 2011. Web. 05 May 2012.
<http://garhildenbrand.com/overview.html>

Shapiro, Rick. "Coley's Toxines". Late Stage Cancer
       2009. Web. 12 May 2012.
 <http://www.latestagecancer.com/2010/04/coleys-
toxins-vaccine-.html>

DAIRY

"Dairy and Diabetes". Personal Interview 2010
<http://www.youtube.com/watch?v=j8FNaOYAJOM>

"Monsanto Cancer Milk". Wilson, S and Akre J.
       Investigative Documentary Video.
<http://www.youtube.com/watch?v=gVKvzHWuJRU>

Wallace, J. "Dairy Products And Cancer." Personal
　　　Interview 2010.
<http://www.youtube.com/watch?v=14ZD-
liw1kQ&lr=1&uid=taVYDVr3RGwxKNdm8nII9g>

Wilson, L. "Epilepsy and Seizures". DrWilson.com
　　　Apr 2011.Web. 13 May 2012.
<http://www.drlwilson.com/articles/epilepsy.htm>

Lane, WM, et al. "The Use of Cow's Milk in Infancy".
　　　Pediatrics 1993. Web. 21 May 2012.
<http://pediatrics.aappublications.org/content/91/2/515.2.abs
tract>

Cohen R. "Say No Way! To Whey!". Dairy Truth 2006. Web. 19
　　　May 2012.
<http://www.dairytruth.com/2006/08/22/say-no-way-to-whey/>

Rietz, D. "Dangers Of Milk And Dairy Products - The
　　　Facts". Rense.com 06 Jul. 2002. Web. 13 May
　　　2012.
<http://www.rense.com/general26/milk.htm>

Gandhi, M. "Milk & diabetes". The Mail Archive 29
　　　Sept. 2005. Web. 13 May 2012.
<http://www.mail-
archive.com/fairfieldlife@yahoogroups.com/msg29997.
html>

Schoffro Cook, M. "Harvard Declares Dairy NOT Part
　　　of a Healthy Diet". Care2 08 Jan 2012. Web. 14
　　　May 2012.
<http://www.care2.com/greenliving/harvard-declares-
dairy-not-part-of-healthy-diet.html>

Food for Breast Cancer . "Milk is not recommended
        for breast cancer". Food for Breast Cancer.
        Web. 13 May 2012.
<http://foodforbreastcancer.com/foods/milk>

Plant, Jane. "Cure Breast Cancer by Avoiding All
        Milk Products". AlkalizeForHealth 24 Jan 2000.
        Web. 13 May 2012.
<http://www.alkalizeforhealth.net/Lnotmilk6.htm>

Ireland, C. "Hormones in Milk Can be Dangerous".
        Harvard U 2006. Web. 26 May 2012.
<http://news.harvard.edu/gazette/2006/12.07/11-
dairy.html>

Plimpton, G. "Not Milk". NotMilk.com. Web. 13 May
        2012.
<http://www.notmilk.com/>

Cowen, Robert. "No Milk: D is for Diabetes". AFH 11
        Dec. 2000. Web. 13 May 2012.
<http://www.alkalizeforhealth.net/Lnotmilk10.htm>

Cohen R. "52 Good reasons to abandon Milk and
        Dairy". NotMilk. Web. 18 May 2012.
<http://www.notmilk.com/52reasons.pdf>

PennState. "Virus kills breast cancer cells in
        laboratory". PennState 22 Sept. 2011. Web 13
        May 2012.
<http://live.psu.edu/story/55260>

DR. ANN WIGMORE

Wigmore, Ann. "Dr. Ann Wigmore's Life Story". Raw
       Living Foods 20 May 2010. Web. 14 May
       2012.
<http://rawlivingfoods.typepad.com/1/2010/05/dr-ann-
wigmores-life-story.html>

OILS, GMO (CANOLA, SOY, CORN, COTTON), MSG, MERCURY, FLUORIDE, CHLORINE, WATER, PROCESSED FOODS

Yiamouyiannis, John. "Fluoride The Silent Killer".
       ConsumerHealth Jan. 1998. Web. 27 May 2012.
<http://www.consumerhealth.org/articles/display.cfm?I
D=19990303222823>

Mercola J. "Warning: This Daily Habit is Bones,
       Brain, Kidneys, and Thyroid". Mercola.com
       Jul. 2010. Web. 27 May 2012
<http://articles.mercola.com/sites/articles/archive/2010/
07/01/paul-connett-interview.aspx>

Mercola J. "Tap Water Toxins: Is Your Water Trying
       to Kill You?". Mercola.com Feb 2009. Web. 27
       May 2012.
<http://articles.mercola.com/sites/articles/archive/2009/
02/05/tap-water-toxins-is-your-water-trying-to-kill-
you.aspx>

Kunin RA. "ABC's of Fluoridation". Drink Your
       Vitamins 2010. Web. 27 May 2012.
<http://www.drinkyourvitamins.com/abcs-of-
fluoridation.html>

Curezone. "Fluoride and Aluminum - toxic
         combination of fluoroaluminum complex".
         Curezone. Web 27 May 2012.
<http://curezone.com/art/read.asp?ID=11&db=12&C0=
12>

Forbes WF and DR McLachlan. "Further thoughts on
         the aluminum-Alzheimer's disease link." NCBI
         Aug. 1996. Web. 27 May 2012.
<http://www.ncbi.nlm.nih.gov/pubmed/8882222>

Fluoride Action Network. "HEALTH EFFECTS:
         Fluoride & the Brain". Fluoride Action Network
         2007. Web. 27 May 2012.
<http://www.fluoridealert.org/health/brain/>

Minton, BL. "New Study Finds Olive Oil Effective
         against HER-2 Breast Cancer". NaturalNews 11
         Jan. 2009. Web. 26 May 2012.
<http://www.naturalnews.com/025290_oil_olive_fat.ht
ml>

Speern, A. "The real truth about Egg Beaters".
         Healthier Talk 21 May 2011. Web 12 May
         2012.
<http://www.healthiertalk.com/real-truth-about-egg-
beaters-3963>

UMMC. "Omega-6 fatty acids". UMMC 2011. Web. 14
         May 2012.
<http://www.umm.edu/altmed/articles/omega-6-
000317.htm>

Tjandrawinata, R, Et al. "Omega-6 fatty acids make prostate cancer cells grow". PSA Rising 1 Aug. 2005. Web. 14 May 2014.
< http://www.psa-rising.com/med/nutrichemo/omega 605.html>

Main, E. "ConAgra Sued for Calling GMO Canola 'Natural'". Rodale 26 Aug. 2011. Web. 14 May 2012.
<http://www.rodale.com/conagra-gmo-lawsuit>

Peskin, Brian. "Fish oil." Personal interview. Audio 2012.
<http://www.brianpeskin.com/>

VIDEO/DOCUMENTARY

TheTruthGirls. Personal interview. 25 Jul. 2010.
<http://www.youtube.com/watch?v=-w9-zYXSMw0>

"The Beautiful Truth". Krocshel, Steve. 2008. Documentary Movie.
<http://articles.mercola.com/sites/articles/archive/20 11/08/14/beautiful-truth-about-outlawed-cancer-treatment.aspx?e_cid=20110814_SNL_Art_1>

ACID REFLUX & FOOD ALLERGY

Davenport, T. "Can a food allergy cause acid reflux?". HealthCentral 20 Jun. 2007. Web. 14 May 2012.
<http://www.healthcentral.com/acid-reflux/c/39/10589/food-acid-reflux?ic=506048>

PH

Rofstad, E, et al. "Acidic extracellular pH promotes Experimental metastasis of human melanoma cells in athymic nude mice." NCBI 2006. Web. 19 May 2012.
<http://www.ncbi.nlm.nih.gov/pubmed/16818644

Balance PH Diet. "Symptoms of Acidosis". Balance PH Diet 2007. Web. 14 May 2012.
<http://www.balance-ph-diet.com/acidosis_symptom.html>

Young, RO. "pH BALANCE: What are the Symptoms of Acidosis?". Alkaline Water Facts 2008. Web. 14 May 2012.
<http://alkaline-water-facts.com/acidosis_symptoms.html>

Frontier.com. "Acidosis". Weight Loss, Health & pH Alkaline Levels 2011. Web. 14 May 2012.
<http://myplace.frontier.com/~felipe2/id9.html>

Puristat. "Why Is a Healthy Pancreas So Vital?". Puristat 2008. Web. 14 May 2012.
<http://www.puristat.com/pancreas/pancreatitis.aspx>

GAD & GABA

BBC News. "Health Diabetes Vaccine Hope". BBC News 14 May 1999. Web . 13 May 2012 .
<http://news.bbc.co.uk/2/hi/health/344105.stm>

Erecinska, M, et al. "Regulation of GABA level in rat brain synaptosomes: fluxes through enzymes of the GABA shunt and effects of glutamate, calcium, and ketone bodies." NCBI 6 Dec 1996. Web 14 May 2012.
<http://www.ncbi.nlm.nih.gov/pubmed/8931464>

Seykans, J. "What is Glutamic Acid Decarboxylase?". LiveStrong 14 Jun 2011. Web. 13 May 2012.
<http://www.livestrong.com/article/304958-what-is-glutamic-acid-decarboxylase/>

DNC News. "GABA: Gamma-Amino Butyric Acid". Denver Naturopathic Clinic. Web. 13 May 2012.
<http://www.denvernaturopathic.com/news/GABA.html>

Various. "gamma-Aminobutyric Acid : biosynthesis". BioInfoBank Library 2012. Web. 13 May 2012.
<http://lib.bioinfo.pl/meid:53696>

NewRx.com. "GAD 67KD antisense leaves colon cancer cells susceptible to cancer therapy." HighBeam 6 Dec 2004. Web. 14 May 2012.
<http://www.highbeam.com/doc/1G1-125727457.html>

Sheldon, AC. "What is The Food Source of Glutamic Acid?". LiveStrong 27 Jan. 2010. Web. 13 May 2012.
<http://www.livestrong.com/article/52055-source-glutamic-acid/>

Seykans, J. "glutamic Acid Decarboxylase". LiveStrong 14 June 2011. Web. 20 May 2012. <http://www.livestrong.com/article/304958-what-is-glutamic-acid-decarboxylase/>

Neuropathic pain

Frazin, N. "Gene Therapy Relieves Neuropathic Pain in Rats". NINDS 31 Jan 2007. Web. 14 May 2012. <http://www.ninds.nih.gov/news_and_events/news_arti cles/news_article_pain_gene_therapy.htm>

Dr. Nicholas Gonzalez

Mercola, J. "A Special Interview with Dr. Nicholas Gonzalez by: Dr. Mercola". Mercola.com 23 Apr. 2011. Web. 11 May 2011. <http://mercola.fileburst.com/PDF/ExpertInterviewTra nscripts/Interview-Gonzalez-on-Alternative-Cancer-Treatments.pdf>

TUMOR ACHES & PAINS (when healing)

Moser, IA. "Healing Testimony: Terminal Breast Cancer". Healing Cancer Naturally Nov 2008. Web. 12 May 2012. <http://www.healingcancernaturally.com/terminal-breastcure-wheatgrass.html>

Toronto Radio Interview. "Interview with Dr. med. Ryke Geerd Hamer". Healing Cancer Naturally 13 March 1999. Web. 13 May 2012. <http://www.healingcancernaturally.com/hamer6.htm l#interview-with-dr-ryke-geerd-hamer-md>

GLUTATHIONE, Curcumin, NAC, EGCG, SAM-e Parkinson's, HIV, IBS, hormones, AI diseases, Anticancer reagents & HIV inhibitors:

JHU. "Reduction of MnO2(birnessite) by Malonic Acid, Acetoacetic Acid, Acetylacetone, And Structurally-Related Compounds". JHU . Wed. 20 May 2012 <https://jscholarship.library.jhu.edu/bitstream/handle/1 774.2/858/Chapter%204%5b1%5d.%20Malonate.pdf?s equence=6>

Wikipidia. "Glutathione". Wikipidia 10 May 2012. Web. 23 May 2012. <http://en.wikipedia.org/wiki/Glutathione>

Jagatha, B, et al. "Curcumin treatment alleviates the effects of glutathione depletion in vitro and in vivo: therapeutic implications for Parkinson's disease explained via in silico studies." NCBI 1 March 2008. Web. 14 May 2012. <http://www.ncbi.nlm.nih.gov/pubmed/18166164>

Santangelo, F. "Intracellular Thiol Concentration Modulating Inflammatory Response: Influence on the Regulation of Cell Functions Through Cysteine Prodrug Approach". Current Medicinal Chemistry, Volume 10, Number 23, December 2003 , pp. 2599-2610(12). Web. 12 May 2012. <http://www.ingentaconnect.com/content/ben/cmc/2003/00000010/00000023/art00012>

Kumaran, VS., et al. "Repletion of antioxidant status by EGCGand retardation of oxidative damage induced macromolecular anomalies in aged rats". ScienceDirect 07 Nov 2007. Web 12 May 2012. <http://www.sciencedirect.com/science/article/pii/S0531556507002495>

Dietz, R. "Glutathione Therapy and Parkinson's Disease". Ezine Articles 05 Aug. 2008. Web. 14 May 2012. <http://ezinearticles.com/?Glutathione-Therapy-and-Parkinsons-Disease&id=1385731>

Yue, P. Et al. "Depletion of intracellular glutathione contributes to JNK-mediated death receptor 5 upregulation and apoptosis induction by the novel synthetic triterpenoid methyl-2-cyano-3,12-dioxooleana-1, 9-dien-28-oate (CDDO-me)". RefDoc 2006. Web. 14 May 2012. <http://cat.inist.fr/?aModele=afficheN&cpsidt=18008398>

Harzenberg, LA, et al. "Glutathione deficiency is associated with impaired survival in HIV disease". PNAS 1997. Web. 15 May 2012. <http://www.pnas.org/content/94/5/1967.full>

Evans, K. "Coconut Oil is The Anti Viral of
        Nature."Natural News 15 Jul. 2009. Web. 24
        June 2012.
<http://www.naturalnews.com/026624_coconut_oil_fat
ty_acids_cleansing.html>

Li, Q, et al. "Glycerol monolaurate prevents mucosal
        SIV transmission." NCBI April 2009. Web. 24
        June 2012.
<http://www.ncbi.nlm.nih.gov/pubmed/19262509>

CconutOil.com. "HIV-AIDS." CoconutOil.Com Web.
        24 June 2012.
<http://coconutoil.com/hiv/>

James, SJ, et al. "Thimerosal Neurotoxicity is
        Associated with Glutathione Depletion:
        Protection with Glutathione Precursors".
        ScienceDirect 29 Sept. 2004. Web. 11 May
        2012
<http://www.sciencedirect.com/science/article/pii/S016
1813X04001147>

Uretsky, S. "Glutathione". Healthline 2005. Web. 13
        May   2012.
<http://www.healthline.com/galecontent/glutathione>

Staffas, L., et al. "Growth hormone- and testosterone-
        dependent regulation of glutathione transferase
        subunit A5 in rat liver." NCBI 15 Jun. 1998.
        Web. May 13, 2012.
<http://www.ncbi.nlm.nih.gov/pmc/articles/PMC1219
538/>

GLUTATHIONE VIDEOS on the "Critical roles that the glutathione molecule performs in every cell in the body (particularly cellular redox homeostasis having to do with maintaining body PH to normal & carrying oxygen to cells):

Nagasawa, H. Personal interview. 26 Dec 2009.
<http://www.youtube.com/watch?v=fYQibc32CfM>

Hyman, Mark. Personal interview. 18 Jul 2008.
<http://www.youtube.com/watch?v=Eh2PYQBICWs>

Amazin-Glutathione. "What Foods have
        Glutathione?" Amazing Glutathione 2009. Web.
        22 May 2012.
<http://www.amazing-glutathione.com/what-foods-have-glutathione.html>

IMMUNOTHERAPY ("treatment of disease by inducing, enhancing, or suppressing an immune response")

Wikipedia. "Immunotherapy." Wikipedia 21June 2012.
        Web. 24 June 2012.
<http://en.wikipedia.org/wiki/Immunotherapy>

INFLAMMATION

Coussens, L, and Z. Werb. "Inflammatory Cells and
        Cancer". NCBI March 2001. Web. 19 May 2012.
<http://www.ncbi.nlm.nih.gov/pmc/articles/PMC2193419/>

Eliaz, Isaac. "Help Your Body Win The Battle Against Autoimmune Disease". Easy Health Options 11 Dec 2011. Web. 03 Jan 2012.
<http://www.easyhealthoptions.com/alternative-medicine/help-your-body-win-the-battle-against-autoimmune-disease/>

KIDNEYS

Chan, A. " Low Carb, high-fat diet could replace dialysis". MSNBC 20 Apr. 2011. Web. 14 May 2012.
<http://www.msnbc.msn.com/id/42689095/ns/health/t/low-carb-high-fat-diet-could-replace-dialysis/>

Fiore, K. "Supplement Averts kidney Stones in Ketogenic Diet". Medpage Today 22 Jul 2009. Web. 16 May 2012.
<http://www.medpagetoday.com/Nephrology/GeneralNephrology/15204>

Barclay, L. "Oral Potassium Citrate May Help Prevent Kidney Stones in Children on the Ketogenic Diet". Medscape 27 Jul 2009. Web. 16 May 2012.
<http://www.medscape.com/viewarticle/706503>

VITAMINS: synthetic vs. Natural nutrients

Nechuta, S., et al. "Vitamin Supplement Use During Breast Cancer Treatment and Survival: A Prospective Cohort Study". NCBI 20 Feb 2011. Web. 13 May 2012.
<http://www.ncbi.nlm.nih.gov/pubmed/21177425>

Chong DH. "Real or Synthetic: The Truth Behind Whole-Food Supplements". Mercola.com 19 Jan. 2005. Web. 26 May 2012.
<http://articles.mercola.com/sites/articles/archive/2005/01/19/whole-food-supplements.aspx>

Mercola J. "Experts Warn: This Popular Vitamin can Trigger Cancer". Mercola.com. 18 Nov. 2011. Web. 26 May 2012.
<http://articles.mercola.com/sites/articles/archive/2011/11/18/dangers-of-vitamins.aspx>

MCP (Modified Citris Pectin), lectins and Galectin-3

VIDEO

Eliaz, I. Personal interview. 15 Sept. 2011.
<http://www.ihealthtube.com/aspx/viewvideo.aspx?v=4e94819a3afdfcfd>

Honjo, Y. et al. "Expression of Cytoplasmic Galectin-3 as a Prognostic Marker in Tongue Carcinoma" Clinical Cancer Research Sep 2000. Web. 14 May 2012.
<http://clincancerres.aacrjournals.org/content/6/12/4635.full>

Medical Dictionary. "Galectin 3". Medical Dictionary 2012. Web. 14 May 2012.
<http://www.medicaldictionaryweb.com/Galectin+3-definition/>

Bartolazzi, A, et al. "Thyroid Cancer Imaging *In Vivo*
By Targeting the Anti-Apoptotic Molecule
Galectin-3". NCBI 2008. Web. 14 May 2012.
<http://www.ncbi.nlm.nih.gov/pmc/articles/PMC2582451/
>

Velmurugan B, et al. "Dietary feeding of grape seed
extract revents intestinal tumorigenesis in
APCmin/+ mice." NCBI Jan. 2010. Web. 16
May 2012.
< http://www.ncbi.nlm.nih.gov/pubmed/20072658>

English, J, and W. Dean. "Modified Citrus Pectin
Inhibition of Cancer Cell Growth and
Metastases". Nutrition
Review 2011. Web. 22 May 2012.
<http://www.nutritionreview.org/library/citrus.pectin.php
>

Hirabayashi, J. "Galectin: Definition and History".
GlycoForum 15 Dec. 1997. Web. 22 May 2012.
<http://www.glycoforum.gr.jp/science/word/lectin/LEA
01E.html>

Klotter, J. "Modified Citrus Pectin- Shorts". Towsend
Letter 2004. Web. 23 May 2012.
<http://findarticles.com/p/articles/mi_m0ISW/is_247-
248/ai_113806990/>

MCP & OTHER DETOX

Eliaz, I. "Guidelines for a Successful Spring Cleanse".
Dr. Eliaz 2011. Web. 23 May 2012.
< http://www.dreliaz.org/blog/guidelines-for-a-successful-spring-cleanse>

Fuchs, NK. "The Amazing Health Benefits of
Modified Citrus Pectin". New Living Magazine
2003. Web 19 May 2012.
<http://www.newliving.com/issues/oct_2003/articles/modified%20citrus%20pectin.html >

COX-2 Inhibitors: QUERCETIN, MCP, RESVERATROL, Vitamin C, Turmeric/Curcumin, melatonin

MedicineNet. "Definition of COX-2". MedicineNet 19
March2012. Web. 23 May 2012.
<http://www.medterms.com/script/main/art.asp?articlekey=7121>

Deng, WG, et al. "Melatonin suppresses macrophage
cyclooxygenase-2 and inducible nitric oxide
synthase expression by inhibiting p52
acetylation and binding". Blood Journal Apr.
2006. Web. 27 May 2012.
<http://bloodjournal.hematologylibrary.org/content/108/2/518.full>

O'Leary KA, et al. "Effect of flavonoids and vitamin E on
cyclooxygenase-2 (COX-2) transcription." NCBI 13
JUL 2004. Web. 16 May 2012.
<http://www.ncbi.nlm.nih.gov/pubmed/15225597>

Goel, A, et al."Specific inhibition of cyclooxygenase-2 (COX-2) expression by dietary curcumin in HT-29 human colon cancer cells." NCBI 30 OCT 2001. Web. 16 May 2012.
<http://www.ncbi.nlm.nih.gov/pubmed/11566484>

Chen CH, et al. "Suppression of endotoxin-induced proinflammatory esponses by citrus pectin through blocking LPS signaling pathways." NCBI OCT 2006. Web. 16 May 2012.
<http://www.ncbi.nlm.nih.gov/pubmed/16930561>

Zykova TA, et al. "Resveratrol Directly Targets COX-2 to Inhibit Carcinogenesis". NCBI OCT 2008. Web. 16 May 2012.
<http://www.ncbi.nlm.nih.gov/pmc/articles/PMC2562941/>

Lee SK, et al. "Vitamin C suppresses proliferation of the human melanoma cell SK-MEL-2 through the inhibition of cyclooxygenase-2 (COX-2) expression and the modulation of insulin-like growth factor II (IGF-II) production." NCBI JUL 2008. Web. 16 May 2012
<http://www.ncbi.nlm.nih.gov/pubmed/18297687>

Gibellini, L. Et al. "Interfering with ROS Metabolism in Cancer Cells: The Potential Role of Quercetin". MDPI 14 Jun 2012. Web. 13 May 2012.
<http://www.mdpi.com/2072-6694/2/2/1288>

Velmurugan B, et al. "Dietary feeding of grape seed extract prevents intestinal tumorigenesis in APCmin/+ mice." NCBI Jan. 2010. Web. 16 May 2012.
< http://www.ncbi.nlm.nih.gov/pubmed/20072658>

METAL

Mannello, F, et al. "Analysis of aluminium content and iron homeostasis in nipple aspirate fluids from healthy women and breast cancer-affected patients." NCBI Apr. 2011. Web. 26 May 2012.
<http://www.ncbi.nlm.nih.gov/pubmed/21337589>

PREGNANCY & ACETONE

Wikipedia. "Acetone". Wikipedia 14 May 2012. Web. 16 May 2012.
<http://en.wikipedia.org/wiki/Acetone>

Campbell. "How I beat cancer". Green Drinks Diaries Oct 2011. Web. 16 May 2012.
<http://www.greendrinkdiaries.com/how-i-beat-cancer/>

Laino, C. "Pregnancy Hormone May Prevent Breast Cancer". FoxNews 20 Apr. 2005. Web. 23 May 2012.
<http://www.foxnews.com/story/0,2933,153964,00.html>

ANGIOGENESIS-PRIMARY TUMOR REMOVED VIA SURGERY GIVE THE CAPACITY TO METASTASIS TO BECOME PRIMARY TUMORS (gets bigger when taken out)

Brunetti ,J. Personal interview. 27 Apr. 2009.
<http://www.myspace.com/video/vid/56502258#pm_cmp=vid_OEV_P_P>

NON GMO & NON HYDROGENATED OILS & CARDIO VASCULAR HEALTH

Perez-Guisado, J., et al. "Spanish Ketogenic
    Mediterranean diet: a healthy cardiovascular
    diet for weight loss"._Nutrition Journal 2008,
    7:30 doi:10.1186/1475-2891-7-30
<http://www.nutritionj.com/content/7/1/30>

Sicar, S, and U. Kansra. "Choice of cooking oils—
    myths and realities". NCBI Oct. 1998. Web. 26
    May 2012.
<http://www.ncbi.nlm.nih.gov/pubmed/10063298>

"The Beautiful Truth". Krocshel, Steve. 2008.
    Documentary Movie.
<http://articles.mercola.com/sites/articles/archive/20
11/08/14/beautiful-truth-about-outlawed-cancer-
treatment.aspx?e_cid=20110814_SNL_Art_1>

ZINC (almonds are a source of zinc)

Nardinocchi, L, et al. "Zinc Downregulates HIG-I and
    Inhibits its Activity in Tumor Celss in Vitro and
    In Vivo." NCBI. Dec. 2010. Web. 20 May 2012.
<http://www.ncbi.nlm.nih.gov/pmc/articles/PMC30014
54/>

Craddock, TJA, et al. "The Zinc Dyshomeostasis
    Hypothesis of Alzheimer's Disease." NCBI. 23
    March 2012. Web. 21 June 2012.
<http://www.ncbi.nlm.nih.gov/pmc/articles/PMC33116
47/?tool=pmcentrez>

ENZYME (Digestive and systemic enzymes)

Wong, W, "The difference Between Systemic and
    Digestive Enzymes." SytemicEnzimes.Net.
    2008. Web. 30 June 2012.
<http://systemicenzymes.net/articles/systemic_vs_diges
tive.html>

Eliaz, Isaac. "Digestive Health." Dr.Eliaz.org. 2011.
    Web. 30 June 2012.
<http://www.dreliaz.org/wellness-guide/digestive-
health>

Return2Health. "The Difference Between Systemic and
    Digestive Enzymes." Return2Health. 2009.
    Web. 30 June 2012.
<http://www.return2health.net/articles/enzyme-
articles/systemic-digestive-enzymes/>

WHEAT/GLUTEN

Allan, Christian B., and Wolfgang Lutz. *Life Without
    Bread.* Los Angeles: Keats Publishing 2000. Print.

Davis, W. *Belly Fat. Rodale Inc. 2011. Print*

JOURNALS

Reimann, SP. "The acid-Base Regulatory Mechanism
in Anesthesia" The American journal of surgery
33 (1919): 86. Web 12 May 2012
<http://books.google.com/books?id=AukAAAAAYAA
J&pg=RA1-
PA86&dq=ketone+increase+alkali&hl=en&ei=J_a-
TvCBAYb20gHM7fiyBA&sa=X&oi=book_result&ct=
result&resnum=2&ved=0CDMQ6AEwAQ#v=onepage
&q=ketone%20increase%20alkali&f=false>

INDEX

CPSIA information can be obtained at www.ICGtesting.com
Printed in the USA
LVOW011323160513

334146LV00005B/35/P